Medical Inquiries and Observations upon the Diseases of the Mind

History of Psychology and Psychiatry

By Benjamin Rush

Professor of the Institutes and Practice of Medicine, and of Clinical Practice, in the University of Pennsylvania

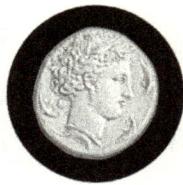

PANTIANOS
CLASSICS

Published by Pantianos Classics

ISBN-13: 978-1-78987-567-6

First published in 1812

This reprint is adapted from the Fourth Edition of 1830

Contents

Disclaimer

Eastern District of Pennsylvania, to wit:

Be it remembered, that on the twenty-sixth day of October, in the thirty-seventh year of the Independence of the United States of America, A. D. 1812, Kimber & Richardson, of the said District, have deposited in this office, the title of a book, the right whereof they claim as proprietors, in the words following, *to wit:-*

"Medical Inquiries and Observations, upon the Diseases of the Mind. By Benjamin Rush, M. D. Professor of the Institutes and Practice of Medicine, and of Clinical Practice, in the University of Pennsylvania."

In conformity to the act of the Congress of the United States, entitled, "An act for the encouragement of learning, by securing the copies of maps, charts, and books, to the authors and proprietors of such copies, during the times therein mentioned." And also to the act, entitled, "An act supplementary to an act, entitled, "An act for the encouragement of learning, by securing the copies of maps, charts, and books, to the authors and proprietors of such copies during the times therein mentioned," and extending the benefits thereof to the arts of designing, engraving, and etching historical and other prints."

D. CALDWELL,
Clerk of the District of Pennsylvania

Preface

Agreeably to a promise made to the public some years ago, and in compliance with the solicitations of the author's pupils, he now offers to them a volume of Medical Inquiries and Observations, upon the Diseases of the Mind.

The views which he has taken of the proximate cause, forms, and symptoms of those diseases, have obliged him to employ a new nomenclature to designate some of them. This becomes no less necessary where new opinions are proposed, or new symptoms described in the history of diseases, than an increase in the number of words, and new combinations of them, become necessary to accompany the increase of the wants and objects of civilized society.

Some of the facts contained in the following pages are of an old date, and will be familiar to the medical reader, but the republication of them, it is hoped will be excused, when it is perceived, that they are placed under the direction of new principles, and that new inferences of a practical nature are deduced from them. An apology may seem necessary likewise for the large number of recent facts that have been added to them. Upon subjects so interesting as the present, more than common testimony is necessary to produce conviction. Besides, facts, or precedents, have the same effects in reasoning in medicine, that examples have in morals. They compel the reader to admit the practice they are intended to establish, provided they are applied in a proper manner.

The author has omitted referring to the books from which he has obtained some of his facts. His reason for doing so was, when he began to collect them, he did not expect to publish them, and of course did not mark the volumes and pages from which they were extracted. Since he formed that design, he has faithfully preserved references to them both. He has suppressed them, only because their partial publication would have destroyed the uniformity of the work. He commits his imperfect labours, now before the reader, to his fellow citizens, with a hope that they may serve as a supplement to materials already collected, from which a system of principles may be formed that shall lead to general success in the treatment of the diseases of the mind. Experience has exhausted herself in abortive efforts for that purpose, and should the following attempt to co-operate with her by principles be alike unsuccessful, it must be ascribed to their being erroneous, for the author believes those diseases can be brought under the dominion of medicine, only by just theories of their seats and proximate cause.

BENJAMIN RUSH

Philadelphia. October 1812.

Chapter One - Of the Faculties and Operations of the Mind, and on the Proximate Cause and Seat of Intellectual Derangement

In entering upon the subject of the following Inquiries and Observations, I feel as if I were about to tread upon consecrated ground. I am aware of its difficulty and importance, and I thus humbly implore that being, whose government extends to the thoughts of all his creatures, so to direct mine, in this arduous undertaking, that nothing hurtful to my fellow citizens may fall from my pen, and that this work may be the means of lessening a portion of some of the greatest evils of human life.

Before I proceed to consider the diseases of the mind, I shall briefly mention its different faculties and operations.

Its faculties are, understanding, memory, imagination, passions, the principle of faith, will, the moral faculty, conscience, and the sense of Deity.

Its principal operations, after sensation, are perception, association, judgment, reasoning and volition. All its subordinate operations, which are known by the names of attention, reflection, contemplation, wit, consciousness, and the like, are nothing but modifications of the five principal operations that have been mentioned.

The faculties of the mind have been called, very happily, *internal* senses. They resemble the external senses in being innate, and depending wholly upon bodily impressions to produce their specific operations. These impressions, are made through the medium of the external senses. As well might we attempt to excite thought in a piece of marble by striking it with our hand, as expect to produce a single operation of the mind in a person deprived of the external senses of touch, seeing, hearing, taste, and smell,

All the operations in the mind are the effects of motions previously excited in the brain, and every idea and thought appears to depend upon a motion peculiar to itself. In a sound state of the mind these motions are regular, and succeed impressions upon the brain with the same certainty and uniformity that perceptions succeed impressions upon the senses in their sound state.

In inquiring into the causes of the diseases of the mind, and the remedies that are proper to relieve them, I shall employ the term derangement to signify the diseases of all the faculties of the mind.

As the understanding occupies the highest rank of those faculties, and as it is most frequently the seat of derangement, I shall begin by considering the causes, and all the states and forms of its diseases.

By derangement in the understanding I mean every departure of the mind in its perceptions, judgments, and reasonings from its natural and habitual order, accompanied with corresponding actions. It differs from delirium, whether acute, or chronic, in being accompanied with a departure from habitual order, in incoherent conduct, as well as conversation. The latter however is not necessary to constitute intellectual madness, for we sometimes meet with the most incongruous actions without incoherent speech, and we now and then meet with incoherent speech in mad people, in whom the disease does not destroy their habits of regular conduct. This is evinced by the correctness with which they sometimes perform certain mechanical and menial pieces of business. Madness is to delirium what walking in sleep is to dreaming. It is delirium, heightened and protracted by a more active and permanent stimulus upon the brain. [1]

Let it not be supposed that intellectual derangement always affects the understanding exclusively in the manner that has been mentioned. Far from it. Two or more of the faculties are generally brought into sympathy with it, and there are cases in which all the faculties are sometimes deranged in succession, and rotation, and now and then they are all affected at the same time. This occurs most frequently in the beginning of a paroxysm of intellectual madness, but it rarely continues to affect the other faculties of the mind after two or three weeks, or after the liberal use of depleting remedies. Thus fever in its first attack, affects the bowels and nervous system, and in a few days settles down into a disease chiefly of the blood vessels.

Derangement in the understanding has been divided into partial and general. The causes of both are the same. I should proceed immediately to enumerate them, but as the seat, or proximate cause, of a disease is generally the first object of a physician's inquiry on entering a sick room, it shall be the first subject of our consideration in the present inquiry.

1. The most ancient opinion of the proximate cause of intellectual derangement, or what has been called madness is, that it is derived from a morbid state of the liver, and that it discovers itself in a vitiated state of the bile. Hippocrates laid the foundation of this error by his encomium upon Democritus whom he found employed in examining the liver of a dumb animal in order to discover the cause of madness.

2. Madness has been said to be the effect of a disease in the spleen. This viscus is supposed to be affected in a peculiar manner in that grade of madness which has been called hypochondriasis. For many years it was known in England by no other name than the spleen, and even to this day, persons who are affected with it are said to be spleeny, in some parts of the New England states.

3. A late French writer, Dr. Prost, in an ingenious work entitled "Medecine Eclairee par Observation et l'Overture des Corps," has taken pains to prove that madness is the effect of a disease in the intestines, and particularly of their peritoneal coat. The marks of inflammation which appear in the bowels, in persons who have died of madness, have no doubt favoured this opinion; but these morbid appearances as well as all those which are often met with in the liver, spleen, and occasionally in the stomach in persons who have died of madness, are the effects, and not the causes of the disease. They are in-

duced either, 1, by the violent or protracted exercises of the mind attracting or absorbing the excitement of those viscera, and thereby leaving them in that debilitated state which naturally disposes them to inflammation and obstruction. Thus diseases in the stomach induces torpor and costiveness in the alimentary canal. Thus too local inflammation often induces coldness and insensibility in contiguous parts of the body. Or, 2, they are induced by the reaction of the mind from the impressions which produce madness, being of such a nature as to throw its morbid excitement upon those viscera with so much force as to produce inflammation and obstructions in them. That they are induced by one, or by both these causes, I infer from the increased secretion and even discharge of bile which succeed a paroxysm of anger; from the pain in the left side, or spleen, which succeeds a paroxysm of malice or revenge; and from the pain, and other signs of disease in the bowels and stomach which follow the chronic operations of fear and grief. That the disease and disorders of all the viscera that have been mentioned, are the effects, and not the causes of madness, I infer further from their existing for weeks, months and years in countries subject to intermitting fevers, without producing madness, or even the least alienation of mind.

4. Madness it has been said is the effect of a disease in the nerves. Of this, dissections afford us no proofs; on the. contrary, they generally exhibit the nerves after death from madness in a sound state. I object further, to this opinion, that hysteria, which is universally admitted to be seated chiefly in the nerves and muscles, often continues for years, and sometimes during a long life, without inducing madness, or if the mind be alienated for a few minutes in one of its paroxysms, it is only from its bringing the vascular system into sympathy, in which I shall say presently the cause of madness is primarily seated. The reaction of the mind from the impressions which produce hysteria, discovers itself in the bowels, in the kidneys, and in most of the muscular parts of the body.

5, and lastly. Madness has been placed exclusively in the mind. I object to this opinion, 1, because the mind is incapable of any operations independently of impressions communicated to it through the medium of the body. 2, Because there are but two instances upon record of the brain being found free from morbid appearances in persons who have died of madness. One of these instances is related by Dr. Stark, the other by Dr. De Haen. They probably arose from the brain being diseased beyond that grade in which inflammation and its usual consequences take place. Did cases of madness reside exclusively in the mind, a sound state of the brain ought to occur after nearly every death from that disease.

I object to it, 3, because there are no instances of primary affections of the mind, such as grief, love, anger, or despair, producing madness until they had induced some obvious changes in the body, such as wakefulness, a full or frequent pulse, costiveness, a dry skin, and other symptoms of bodily indisposition.

I know it has been said in favour of madness being an ideal disease, or being seated primarily in the mind, that sudden impressions from fear, terror, and even ridicule have sometimes cured it. This is true, but they produce their effects only by the healthy actions they induce in the brain. We see several other diseases, particularly hiccup, head-ache, and even fits of epilepsy, which are evidently affections of the body, cured in the same way by impressions of fear and terror upon the mind.

Having rejected the abdominal viscera, the nerves, and the mind, as the primary seats of madness, I shall now deliver an opinion, which I have long believed and taught in my lectures, and that is, that the cause of madness is seated primarily in the blood-vessels of the brain, and that it depends upon the same kind of morbid and irregular actions that constitute other arterial diseases. There is nothing specific in these actions. They are a part of the unity of disease, particularly of fever; of which madness is a chronic form, affecting that part of the brain which is the seat of the mind.

My reasons for believing the cause of madness to be seated in the blood-vessels of the brain are drawn,

I. From its remote and exciting causes, many of which are the same with those which induce fever and certain diseases of the brain, particularly phrenitis, apoplexy, palsy, and epilepsy, all of which are admitted to have their seats in a greater or less degree in the blood-vessels. Of thirty-six dissections of the brains of persons who had died of madness, Mr. Pinel says he could perceive no difference between the morbid appearances in them, and in the brains of persons who had died of apoplexy and epilepsy. The sameness of these appearances however do not prove that all those diseases occupy the same parts of the brain: I believe they do not, especially in their first stage: they become diffused over the whole brain, probably in their last stages, or in the paroxysm of death. Dr. Johnson, of Exeter, in speaking of the diseases of the abdominal viscera, mentions their sympathy with each other, by what he very happily calls "an intercommunion of sensation." It would seem as if a similar intercommunion took place between all the diseases of the brain. It is remarkable they all discover, in every part of the brain, marks of a morbid state of the blood-vessels.

II. From the ages and constitutions of persons who are most subject to madness. The former are in those years in which acute and inflammatory arterial diseases usually affect the body, and the latter, in persons who labour under the arterial predisposition.

III. I infer that madness is seated in the blood vessels,

1. From its symptoms. These are a sense of fulness, and sometimes pain in the head; wakefulness, and a redness of the eyes, such as precede fever, a whitish tongue, a dry or moist skin, high coloured urine, a frequent, full, or tense pulse, or a pulse morbidly slow or natural as to frequency. These states of the pulse occur uniformly in recent madness, and one of them, that is frequency, is seldom absent in its chronic state.

I have taken notice of the presence of this symptom in my Introductory Lecture upon the Study of Medical Jurisprudence, in which I have mentioned, that seven-eighths of all the deranged patients in the Pennsylvania Hospital in the year 1811 had frequent pulses, [2] and that a pardon was granted to a criminal by the president of the United States, in the year 1794, who was suspected of counterfeiting madness, in consequence of its having been declared by three physicians that that symptom constituted an unequivocal mark of intellectual derangement.

The connection of this disease with the state of the pulse has been further demonstrated by a most satisfactory experiment, made by Dr. Coxe, and related by him in his Practical Observations upon Insanity. He gave digitalis to a patient who was in a furious state of madness, with a pulse that beat 90 strokes in a minute. As soon as the medicine reduced his pulse to 70, he became rational. Upon continuing it, his pulse fell to 50, at which time he became melancholy. An additional quantity of the medicine reduced it to 40 strokes in a minute, which nearly suspended his life. He was finally cured by lessening the doses of the medicine so as to elevate his pulse to 70 strokes in a minute, which was probably its natural state. In short there is not a single symptom that takes place in an ordinary fever, except a hot skin, that does not occur in the acute state of madness.

IV. From its alternating with several diseases which are evidently seated in the blood-vessels. These are consumption, rheumatism, intermitting and puerperal fever, and dropsy, many instances of which are to be met with in the records of medicine.

V. From its blending its symptoms with several of the forms of fever. It is sometimes attended with regular intermissions, and remissions. I have once seen it appear with profuse sweats, such as occur in certain fevers, in a madman in the Pennsylvania Hospital. These sweats, when discharged from his skin, formed a vapour resembling a thick fog, that filled the cell in which he was confined to such a degree as to render his body scarcely visible.

Again, this disease sometimes appears in a typhus form, in which it is attended with coldness, a feeble pulse, muttering delirium, and involuntary discharge of fasces and urine. But it now and then pervades a whole country in the form of an epidemic. It prevailed in this way in England in the years 1355 and 1373, and in France and Italy in the year 1374, and Dr. Wintringham mentions its frequent occurrence in England in the year 1719.

A striking instance of the union of madness with common fever is mentioned by Lucian. He tells us that a violent fever once broke out at Abdera, which terminated by hemorrhages, or sweats, on the seventh day. During the continuance of this fever the patients affected with it, repeated passages from the tragedy of Andromeda with great vehemence, both in their sick rooms and in the public streets. This mixture of fever and madness continued until the coming on of cold weather. Lucian ingeniously and very properly ascribes it to the persons affected, having heard the famous player Archilaus act a part in the above tragedy in the middle of summer, in so impressive a manner that it excited in them the seeds of a dormant fever which blended itself with derangement, and thus produced, very naturally, a repetition of the ideas and sounds that excited their disease.

VI. From the appearances of the blood which is drawn in this disease being the same as that which is drawn in certain fevers. They are, inflammatory buff, yellow, serum, and lotura carnium.

VII. From the appearances of the brain after death from madness. These are nearly the same as after death from phrenitis, apoplexy, and other diseases which are admitted to be primary affections of the blood-vessels of the brain. I shall briefly enumerate them; they are, 1, the absence of every sign of disease. I have ascribed this to that grade of suffocated excitement which prevents tlv effusion of red blood into the serous vessels. We observe the same absence of the marks of inflammation after several other violent diseases. Dr. Stevens in his ingenious inaugural dissertation published in 1811, has called this apparently healthy appearance, the "aimatous" state of inflammation. Perhaps it would be more proper to call it the "aimatous" state of disease. It is possible it may arise in *recent* cases of madness which terminate fatally, from the same retrocession of the blood from the brain which takes place from the face and external surface of the body, just before death. But,

2. We much oftener discover in the brain, after death from madness, inflammation, effusions of water in its ventricles, extravasation and intravation of blood, and even pus. After chronic madness, we discover some peculiar appearances which have never been met with in any other disease of the brain, and these are a preternatural hardness, and dryness in all its parts. Lieutaud mentions it often with the epithets of "durum," "praedurum," "siccum," and "exsuccum." Morgagni takes notice of this hardness likewise, and says he had observed it in the cerebrum in persons in whom the cerebellum retained its natural softness. Dr. Bailie and Mr. John Hunter have remarked, that the brain in this state discovered marks of elasticity when pressed by the fingers. Mr. Mickell says a cube of six lines of the brain of a maniac, thus indurated, weighed seven drams, whereas a cube of the same dimension of a sound brain weighed but one dram, and between four and six grains. I have ascribed this hardness, dryness, elasticity and relative weight of the brain to a tendency to schirrus, such as succeeds morbid action or inflammation in glandular parts of the body, and particularly that early grade of it which occurs in the liver, and which is known by the name of hepitalgia. The brain in this case loses its mobility so as to become incapable of emitting those motions from impressions which produce the operations of the mind.

3. We sometimes discover preternatural softness in the brain, in persons who die of madness, similar to that which we find in other viscera from common and febrile diseases. This has been observed to occur most frequently in the kidneys and spleen. The brain in this case partakes of its tex-

ture and imbecility in infancy, and hence its inability to receive, and modify the impressions which excite thought in the mind.

4. and lastly. We sometimes discover a preternatural enlargement of the bones of the head from madness, and sometimes a preternatural reduction of their thickness. Of 216 maniacs, whose heads were examined, after death, Dr. Creighton says in 160 the skull was enlarged, and in 38 it was reduced in its thickness. Now the same thing succeeds rheumatism, and many other febrile diseases which exert their action in the neighbourhood of bones.

I might add further, under this head, that the morbid appearances in the spleen, liver, and stomach, which are seen after death from madness, place it still more upon a footing with fevers from all its causes, and particularly from koino-miasmatic exhalations, and in a more especial manner when they affect the brain, and thereby induce primary, or idiopathic phrenitis. In short madness is to phrenitis, what pulmonary consumption is to pneumony, that is a chronic state of an acute disease. It resembles pulmonary consumption further, in the excitement of the muscles, and in the appetite continuing in a natural, or in a preternatural state.

VIII. I infer madness to be primarily seated in the blood-vessels, from the remedies which most speedily and certainly cute it, being exactly the same as those which cure fever or disease in the blood-vessels from other causes, and in other parts of the body. They will be noticed in their proper place.

I have thus mentioned the facts and arguments which prove what is commonly called madness to be a disease of the blood-vessels of the brain. All the other and inferior forms of derangement, whether of the memory, the will, the principle of faith, the passions, and the moral faculties, I believe to be connected more or less with morbid action in the blood-vessels of the brain, or heart, according to the seats of those faculties of the mind.

In placing the primary seat of madness in the blood-vessels, I would by no means confine the predisposition to it exclusively to them. It extends to the nerves, and to that part of the brain which is the seat of the mind, both of which when preternaturally irritable, communicate more promptly, deranged action to the blood-vessels of the brain. I have called the union of this diffused morbid irritability, the phrenitic predisposition. It is from the constant presence of this predisposition, that some people are seldom affected with the slightest fever, without becoming delirious; and it is from its absence, that many people are affected with fevers and other diseases of the brain, without being affected with derangement. I am aware that it may be objected to the proximate cause or seat of madness, which has been delivered, that dissections have sometimes discovered marks of arterial diseases in the brain similar to those that have been mentioned, which were not preceded by the least alienation of mind. In these cases, I would suppose the diseases may have existed in parts of the brain which are not occupied by the mind, or that the mind may have been translated to another, and a healthy part of the brain. The senses of taste and hearing, we know, when impaired by disease, are often translated to contiguous, and sometimes to remote parts of the body. But did we admit the objection that I have met, to militate against madness being an arterial disease, it would prove too much, for we sometimes discover the same morbid appearances, which produce apoplexy and palsy, to be present in the brain after death, without any of the common symptoms of those diseases having been preceded by them.

Many other organic diseases are occasionally devoid of their usual characteristic symptoms. Neither vomiting, nor want of appetite, have taken place in stomachs in which mortification has been discovered after death; and abscesses have been found in the livers of persons, who have died without any one of the common symptoms of hepatitis. By allowing the same latitude to the "confused and irregular operations of nature," in the brain, in the production of madness, that we observe in the production of all the other diseases that have been mentioned, we can reconcile its occasional absence, with the existence of all the organic affections in the brain which usually produce it.

In reviewing the numerous proofs of madness, being seated primarily in the blood-vessels, and its being accompanied so generally with most of the symptoms of fever, we cannot help being struck with the histories of the disease that have been given by many ancient and modern physicians. Galen, defines it to be "delirium sine febre." Aritaeus says it is "semper sine febre." Dr. Arnold quotes a group of authors, who have adopted and propagated the same error. Even Dr. Heberden admits and reasons upon it. The antiquity and extent of this error should lead us never to lose sight of the blood-vessels in investigating the causes of diseases. They are, to a physician, what the meridian sun is to a mariner. There are but few diseases in which it will be possible for him to preserve the system in a healthy course, without daily, and often more frequent observations of the state of the blood-vessels, as manifested by the different and varying states of the pulse.

[1] The reader will find several other distinguishing marks between madness and delirium, applicable to legal purposes, in the author's Introductory Lecture upon Medical Jurisprudence, published in a volume of Lectures, by Bradford and Inskeep, in the year 1810.
[2] This fact was ascertained, at my request, with great accuracy, by Dr. Frederick Vandyke. It is probable the pulsations of the arteries in the brain were preternaturally frequent in the brain in the few cases in which they were natural at the wrists. Dr. Cox, of Bristol, informs us that he had found the carotid artery to be full and tense, when the radial artery was weak and soft.

Chapter Two - Of the remote and exciting causes of intellectual derangement

I have combined both these classes of causes, inasmuch as they most commonly act in concert, or in a natural succession to each other. In enumerating them, I shall include such as act alike in producing partial and universal madness.

They have been divided, 1, into such as act, *directly* upon the body; and, 2, such as act *indirectly* upon the body, through the medium of the mind.

To the first head belongs, 1, all those causes which act *directly* upon the brain. These are, 1, malconformation and laesions of the brain. Between the latter, and the existence of madness, there is sometimes an interval of several years. A young man died in the Pennsylvania Hospital in the year 1809, who became deranged at twenty-one, in consequence of a contusion on his head by a fall from a horse in the fifteenth year of his age. A Mr. ___ died of madness in the same place, from an injury done to his brain by being thrown out of his chair, between two and three years before he discovered any signs of derangement. It is remarkable that injuries show themselves more slowly in the brain than in other parts of the body. Dr. Lettsom mentions a case, in the Memoirs of the London Medical Society, of a disease in the brain, induced by a fall from a horse, which did not discover itself until two and twenty years after its occurrence.

2. Certain local disorders, induced by enlargement of bone, tumors, abscesses, and water in the brain.

3. Certain diseases of the brain, particularly apoplexy, palsy, epilepsy, vertigo, and headache. It occurs but rarely from the last of those causes.

4. Insolation. Two cases of madness from this cause occurred under my care between July 1807, and February 1808.

5. Certain odours. There is a place in Scotland where madness is sometimes induced by the fumes of lead. Patients who are affected with it bite their hands, and tear their flesh upon the other parts of their bodies. It is called by the country people mill-reck. Dr. Prost describes a furious grade of madness in Peru, brought on by a mineral exhalation, but he does not mention the metal from which it is derived. From among many other facts that might be mentioned, to show the connection of odours with a morbid state of the mind, I shall mention one more. An ingenious dyer, in this city, informed me that he often observed the men who were employed in dying blue, of which colour indigo is the basis, to become peevish, and low spirited, and never even to hum a tune, while engaged at their work.

There are certain causes which induce madness, by acting upon the brain in common with the *whole* body. These are, 1, gout, dropsy, consumption, pregnancy, and fevers of all kinds.

2. Inanition from profuse evacuations, or from a defect of nourishment. Famine induces it in part from the latter cause.

3. The sudden abstraction of the stimulus of distension. When madness follows parturition, it is most commonly derived from this cause.

4. The excessive use of ardent spirits. During the time Dr. Nicholas Waters acted as resident physician and apothecary of the Pennsylvania Hospital, he instituted an inquiry at my request, into the proportion of maniacs from this cause, who were confined in the Hospital. They amounted to one-third of the whole number.

5. Inordinate sexual desires and gratifications. Several cases of madness from this cause have come under my notice.

6. Onanism. Four cases of madness occurred, in my practice, from this cause, between the years 1804 and 1807. It is induced more frequently by this cause in young men, than is commonly supposed by parents and physicians. The morbid effects of intemperance in a sexual intercourse with women are feeble, and of a transient nature, compared with the train of physical and moral evils which this solitary vice fixes upon the body and mind.

7. The transfusion of blood from one animal into the blood-vessels of another. This practice was employed in France many years ago, in order to discover a method of restoring health, and renovating life, in sick and aged people. All the persons, Dionis tells us, who were the subjects of it, died in a state of derangement. The practice was founded in error; for old age and sickness are occasioned by exhausted or diseased solids, and not by any unfitness in the quality of the blood, to support animal life.

8. Great pain.

9. Unusual labour or exercise.

10. Extremely hot and cold weather.

3. Madness is induced by corporeal causes, which act *sympathetically* upon the bruin. These are, 1, certain narcotic substances, particularly opium, hemlock, night-shade, henbane, and acconitum, taken into the stomach.

2. The suppression of any usual evacuation, such as the menses, lochia, milk, semen, or blood from the hemorrhoidal vessels.

3. Worms in the alimentary canal.

4. Irritation from certain foreign matters retained in irritable parts of the body. I once knew some small shot which were lodged in the foot of a school boy, induce madness several years after he became a man. It has been brought on in one instance by decayed teeth, which were not accompanied with pain.

4. Madness is sometimes induced by what is called a *metastasis* of some other disease to the brain. These diseases are, 1, dropsy. A case of madness from this cause is related by Dr. Mead. 2. Consumption. All the symptoms of this disease sometimes suddenly disappear, in consequence of the translation of morbid excitement to the brain.

3. St. Vitus's dance. I attended a young lady some years ago, in whom this disease was suspended by an attack of madness. Her madness passed out of her brain, through the same channel by which it entered it, that is, in convul-

16

sions in the limbs of one side, which gradually yielded to the power of medicine.

4. Hysteria. The morbid commotions in the nervous system are sometimes transferred to the blood-vessels, and the brain, where they induce transient or chronic madness.

5. Certain cutaneous eruptions. The son of Dr. Zimmerman became deranged in consequence of an eruption being repelled from his skin. I attended a private patient in the Pennsylvania Hospital, in whom madness was induced by the same cause. The healing of an old and habitual ulcer, has sometimes produced the same effect.

6. The measles. A young man, of sixteen years of age, was admitted into the Pennsylvania Hospital, in June 1812, in a high state of derangement, which followed this disease.

II. The causes which induce intellectual derangement, by acting upon the body through the medium of the mind, are of a direct and indirect nature.

The causes which act directly upon the understanding are,

1. Intense study, whether of the sciences or of the mechanical arts, and whether of real or imaginary objects of knowledge. The latter more frequently produce madness than the former. They are, chiefly, the means of discovering perpetual motion; of converting the base metals into gold; of prolonging life to the antediluvian age; of producing perfect order and happiness in morals and government, by the operations of human reason; and, lastly, researches into the meaning of certain prophesies in the Old and New Testaments. I think I have observed madness from the last cause, to arise most frequently from an attempt to fix the precise time in which those prophesies were to be fulfilled, or from a disappointment in that time, after it had passed.

2. The frequent and rapid transition of the mind from one subject to another. It is said booksellers have sometimes become deranged from this cause. The debilitating effects of these sudden transitions upon the mind, are sensibly felt after reading a volume of reviews or magazines. The brain in these cases is deprived of the benefit of habit, which prevents fatigue to a certain extent, from all the exercises of the body and mind, when they are confined to single objects.

It is worthy of notice that this cause of madness accords exactly with a symptom of one of its forms, and that is, a constant and rapid transition of the mind to a variety of unrelated subjects. But the understanding is affected chiefly in an *indirect* manner.

1. Through the medium of the imagination. It is conveyed into the understanding from this faculty, in all those people who become deranged from inordinate schemes of ambition or avarice. Mad-houses, in every part of the world, exhibit instances of persons who have become insane from this cause. The great extent and constant exercises of the imagination in poets, accounts for their being occasionally affected with this disease.

2. The understanding is sometimes affected with madness through the medium of the memory. Dr. Zimmerman relates the case of a Swiss clergyman, in whom derangement was induced by undue labour in committing his sermons to memory.

3. But madness is excited in the understanding most frequently by impressions that act primarily upon the heart. I shall enumerate some of these impressions, and afterwards mention such instances of their morbid effects as I have met with in the course of my reading and observations. They are joy, terror, love, fear, grief, distress, shame from offended delicacy, defamation, calumny, ridicule, absence from native country, the loss of liberty, property, and beauty, gaming, and inordinate love of praise, domestic tyranny, and, lastly, the complete gratification of every wish of the heart.

Extravagant joy produced madness in many of the successful adventurers in the South Sea speculation in England, in the year 1720.

Charles the Sixth, of France, was deranged from a paroxysm of anger.

Terror has often induced madness in persons who have escaped from fire, earthquakes, and shipwreck. Two cases from the last cause have occurred under my notice.

Where is the mad-house that does not contain patients from neglected, or disappointed love?

Fear often produces madness, Dr. Brambiila tells us, in new recruits in the Austrian army.

Grief induced madness which continued fifty years, in a certain Hannah Lewis, formerly a patient in the Pennsylvania Hospital.

Distress often produced this disease, Mr. Howard tells us, in the prisoners of the town of Liege.

An exquisite sense of delicacy, Dr. Burton says, produced madness in a schoolmaster, who Was accidentally discovered upon a close-stool by one of his scholars.

The Bedlams of Europe exhibit many cases of madness from public and private defamation, and history informs us of ministers of state and generals of armies having often languished away their lives in a state of partial derangement, in consequence of being unjustly dismissed by their sovereigns.

A player destroyed himself in Philadelphia, in the year 1803, soon after being hissed off the stage.

The Swiss soldiers sometimes languish and die from that form of madness which is brought on by absence from their native country.

An ingenious modern poet mentions this disease, as well as its exciting cause, with peculiar elegance.

"The intrepid Swiss that guards a foreign shore,
"Condemn'd to climb his mountain-cliffs no more,
"If chance he hear the song, so sweetly wild,
"Which, on those cliffs, his infant hours beguil'd,
"Melts at the long lost scenes that round him rise,

18

"And sinks, a martyr to repentant sighs."

It is remarkable, this disease is most commonly among the natives of countries that are the least desirable for beauty, fertility, climate, or the luxuries of life. They resemble in this respect, in their influence upon the human heart, the artificial objects of taste which are at first disagreeable, but which from habit take a stronger hold upon the appetite than such as are natural and agreeable.

The Africans become insane, we are told, in some instances, soon after they enter upon the toils of perpetual slavery in the West Indies,

Hundreds have become insane in consequence of unexpected losses of money. It is remarkable this disease occurs oftener among the rich who lose only a part of their property, than among persons in moderate circumstances, who lose their all.

An American Indian became deranged, and destroyed himself, in consequence of seeing his face in a looking glass soon after his recovery from a violent attack of the small-pox. The loss of one eye, by an affray in a country tavern, which materially affected the beauty of the face, produced derangement in a young man who was afterwards my patient in the Pennsylvania Hospital. There are other facts, which show the depth of this attachment to beauty in the human mind, and the poignancy of the distress occasioned by its loss, or decay. The once beautiful lady Mary Wortley Montague tells a friend, in one of her letters, that she had not seen herself in a looking glass for eleven years, solely from her inability to bear the mortifying contrast between her appearance in the two extremes of her life.

A clergyman in Maryland became insane in consequence of having permitted some typographical errors to escape in a sermon which he published upon the death of general Washington.

The son of a late celebrated author in England became deranged in consequence of the severe treatment he received from his father in the course of his education. Several instances of madness, induced by the cruel or unjust conduct of school masters and guardians to the persons who were the subjects of their power and care, are to be met with in the records of medicine.

Sir Philip Mordaunt shot himself immediately after succeeding to a great estate, and to the favour of his prince, and while he appeared to be in possession of every thing that could constitute the plenitude of human happiness. The eldest son of a Scotch nobleman, of high rank and large fortune, destroyed himself in the same way, a few weeks after the consummation of all his worldly prospects and enjoyments by his marriage to a most accomplished and amiable young lady.

Two instances are upon record, of persons who destroyed themselves immediately after drawing high prizes in a lottery. In all these cases death was the effect of derangement.

4. The understanding is sometimes deranged through the medium of the moral faculties. A conscience burdened with guilt, whether real or imaginary,

is a frequent cause of madness. The latter produces it much oftener than the former.

An instance of insanity occurred in a married woman in this city some years ago, of the most exemplary character, from a belief that she had been unfaithful to the marriage bed. An accident discovered that the supposed criminal connection was with a man whose very person was unknown to her. There is further a morbid sensibility in the conscience in some people, that predisposes to madness from the most trifling causes. A young man, of great piety, died of this disease in our Hospital a few years ago, in consequence of his believing that he had offended his Maker by refusing to say grace at the table of a friend.

The most distressing grade of derangement under this head is, where real guilt, and a diseased imagination, concur in producing it. The occasional acts of self-mutilation which deranged patients sometimes inflict upon them-selves, and the painful and protracted austerities voluntarily imposed upon the body in Catholic countries, appear to be the effects of the combined oper-ation of these two causes upon the understanding.

But we sometimes observe intellectual derangement to occur from the moral faculties being unduly excited by supposed visions and revelations, instances of which will be mentioned in another place.

Let not religion be blamed for these cases of insanity. The tendency of all its doctrines and precepts is to prevent it from most of its mental causes; and even the errors that have been blend with it produce madness less frequent-ly than love, and many of those common and necessary pursuits, which con-stitute the principal enjoyments and business of life.

To the history of the causes of derangement which has been given, I shall add, that that form of it which has been called hypochondriasis, is sometimes induced without either the patient or his friends being able to ascribe it to any cause. Dr. Nicholas Robinson, a physician who lived in the beginning of the last century, complains, in a treatise which he has published upon melan-choly, of his sufferings from it in the following words: "When no air has blown across my affairs, and no shade obscured my sun, then am I most mis-erable." I have heard similar declarations from several of my patients, and particularly from a clergyman of the most exemplary life and conversation. In all such cases it would be absurd to suppose the disease existed without a cause. Many diseases take place in the body from causes that are forgotten, or from sympathies with parts of the body that are supposed to be in a healthy state. In like manner, depression of mind may be induced by causes that are forgotten, or by the presence of objects which revive the sensation of distress with which it was at one time associated, but without reviving the cause of it in the memory. The former pupils of the author will recollect sev-eral instances of mental pleasure, as well as pain, from association, men-tioned by him in his physiological lectures upon the mind, in which the origi-nal causes of both had perished in the memory.

Intellectual derangement is more common from mental, than corporeal causes. Of 113 patients in the Bicetre Hospital, in France, at one time, Mr. Pinel tells us 34 were from domestic misfortunes, 24 from disappointments in love, 30 from the distressing events of the French Revolution, and 25 from what he calls fanaticism, making in all the original number, I have taken pains to ascertain the proportion of mental and corporeal causes which have operated in producing madness in the Pennsylvania Hospital, but I am sorry to add, my success in this inquiry was less satisfactory than I wished. Its causes were concealed in some instances, and forgotten in others. Of 50 maniacs, the causes of whose disease were discovered by Dr. Moore and his assistant Mr. Jenny, in the month of April 1812, 7 were from disappointments, chiefly in love; 7 from grief; 7 from the loss of property; 5 from erroneous opinions in religion; 2 from jealousy; 1 from terror; 1 from insolation; 1 from an injury to the head; 2 from repelled eruptions; 5 from intemperance; 3 from onanism; 2 from pregnancy; and 1 from fever; making in all 34 from mental, and 16 from corporeal causes. A predisposition to the disease was hereditary in but five of them,

I shall now mention all those circumstances in birth, certain peculiarities of the body, age, sex, condition and rank in life, intellect, occupation, climate, state of society, forms of government, revolutions, and religion, which *predispose* the body and mind to be acted upon by the remote and exciting causes that have been mentioned, so as to favour the production of madness.

I. A peculiar and hereditary sameness of organization of the nerves, brain, and blood-vessels, on which I said formerly the predisposition to madness depended, sometimes pervades whole families, and renders them liable to this disease from a transient or feeble operation of its causes.

Application was made some years ago for the admission of three members of the same family into the Pennsylvania Hospital on the same day. I have attended two ladies, one of whom was the fourth, and the other the ninth, of their respective families, that had been affected with this disease in two generations.

The following letter to the author, from Dr. Stephen W. Williams, of Deerfield, in Massachusetts, contains the history of two cases of hereditary madness, which, from the singular resemblance in their subjects, symptoms, and issue, have seldom perhaps been met with in the records of medicine.

June 16th, 1812.

Dear Sir,

"Believing that 'the science of medicine is related to every thing,' I am induced to transmit to you the following incidents which have lately occurred in the vicinity of this place, hoping that some useful inductions may be drawn from them, for the benefit of our profession.

"Captains C. L. and J. L. were twin brothers, and so great was the similarity in their countenances and appearance, that it was extremely difficult for strangers to know them apart. Even their friends were often deceived by them. Their habits and manners were likewise similar. Many ludicrous stories are told of people mistaking one for the other.

"They both entered the American revolutionary army at the same time. Both held similar commissions, and both served with honour during the war. They were cheerful, sociable, and in every respect gentlemen. They were happy in their families, having amiable wives and children, and they were both independent in their property. Some time after the close of the war, captain J. removed to the state of Vermont, while captain C. remained in Greenfield, in the vicinity of Deerfield, and 200 miles from his brother. Within the course of three years, they have both been subject to turns of partial derangement, but by no means rising into mania, nor sinking into melancholy. They appeared to be hurried and confused in their manners, but were constantly able to attend to their business. About two years ago, captain J. on his return from the general assembly of Vermont, of which he was a member, was found in his chamber, early in the morning, with his throat cut, by his own hand, from ear to ear, shortly after which he expired. He had been melancholy a few days previous to this fatal catastrophe, and had complained of indisposition the evening previous to the event.

"About ten days ago, captain C. of Greenfield, discovered signs of melancholy, and expressed a fear that he should destroy himself. Early in the morning of June fifth he got up, and proposed to his wife to take a ride with him. He shaved himself as usual, wiped his razor, and stepped into an adjoining room, as his wife supposed, to put it up. Shortly after she heard a noise, like water or blood running upon the floor. She hurried into the room, but was too late to save him. He had cut his throat with his razor, and soon afterwards expired.

"The mother of these two gentlemen, an aged lady, is now in a state of derangement, and their two sisters, the only survivors of their family, have been subject, for several years, to the same complaint."

There are several peculiarities which attend this disease, where the predisposition to it is hereditary, which deserve our notice.

1. It is excited by more feeble causes than in persons in whom this predisposition has been acquired.

2. It generally attacks in those stages of life in which it has appeared in the patient's ancestors. A general officer, who served in the American army during the revolutionary war, once expressed a wish to a brother officer, from whom I received the information, "that he might not live to be old, that he might die suddenly, and that if he married, he might have no issue." Upon being asked the reason for these wishes, he said, he was descended from a family in which madness had sometimes appeared about the fiftieth year of life, and that he did not wish to incur the chance of inheriting, and propagating it to a family of children. He was gratified in all his three wishes. He fell in battle between the thirtieth and fortieth years of his age, and he left no issue, although he had been married several years before his death. A similar in-

stance of the disease appearing at the same time of life, in three persons of the same family, occurred under my notice in the Pennsylvania Hospital. It came on in a father and two of his sons between the sixtieth and seventieth years of their lives.

3. Children born previously to the attack of madness in their parents are less liable to inherit it than those who are born after it.

4. Dr. Burton, in his Anatomy of Melancholy, remarks, that children born of parents who are in the decline of life, are more predisposed to one of the forms of partial insanity than children born under contrary circumstances.

5. A predisposition to certain diseases seated in parts contiguous to the seat of madness, often descends from parents to their children. - Thus we sometimes see madness in a son whose father or mother had been afflicted only with hysteria, or habitual head-ache. The reverse of this remark likewise sometimes takes place. I attended a respectable mechanic in this city in two attacks of madness, the last of which terminated his life. All his children, six in number, and now all adults, are afflicted with head-ache, but none of them have ever discovered any sign of madness in their conduct or conversation.

6. There are instances of families in which madness has existed, where the disease has passed by the understanding in their posterity, and appeared in great strength and excentricity of the memory, and of the passions, or in great perversion of their moral faculties. Sometimes it passes by all the faculties of the mind, and appears only in the nervous system, in persons descended from deranged parents, and again we see madness in children whose parents were remarkable only for eccentricity of mind.

There are several diseases which attack the children of the same family, which did not exist in their ancestors. I have called them filial diseases. They are chiefly consumption and epilepsy. I have attempted to discover whether madness ever appears in this way, and have heard of but two instances of it. One of them occurred in a family in the island of Barbadoes, in which four children, descended from parents of habitually sound minds, became deranged. Perhaps in these cases the disease had existed in their remote ancestors, or possibly it was translated from a disease in some of the contiguous systems of the body. I have wished to discover whether there be any peculiarity of shape in the skulls of mad people that predisposed to derangement, for which purpose I requested Dr. Vandyke, in the year 1810, to examine the dimensions of the heads of all the insane patients in our hospital in several different directions, and afterwards to measure in the same way the heads of a number of patients, belonging to the Hospital, with other diseases. The result of this inquiry was a discovery that there was no departure but in one instance from the ordinary and natural shape of the head, in between sixty and seventy mad people.

II. A predisposition to madness is said to be connected with dark coloured hair. Mr. Haslam informs us that this was the case in two hundred and five out of two hundred and sixty-five patients in the Bethlehem Hospital. He intimates that it was possibly from their consisting chiefly of the natives of England, in whom that colour of the hair is very general; but the same connection between madness and dark coloured hair has been discovered in the maniacs in the Pennsylvania Hospital, who consist of persons from three or four different countries, or of descendants who inherit their various physical characters. Of nearly seventy patients, who were examined at my request, by Dr. Vandyke, in our Hospital, in the year 1810, with a reference to this fact, all, except one, had dark coloured hair. In the month of April, 1812, I requested Dr. Vandyke to direct his inquiries more particularly to the colour of the eyes in the maniacal patients in our Hospital. He executed my request with great care and correctness, and discovered that fifty-six out of seventy-nine of them had light coloured eyes, of which number but six had fair hair.

III. There is a greater predisposition to madness between twenty and fifty, than in any of the previous or subsequent years of human life. Of the correctness of this remark, Mr. Pinel has furnished us with the following proof. Of 1201 persons who were admitted into the Bicetre Hospital, in France, between the years 1784 and 1794, 955 were between the two ages that have been mentioned. 65 were between fifteen and twenty, 131 were between fifty and sixty, and 51 between sixty and seventy-one. Mr. Haslam has furnished additional evidence of the correctness of this remark. Of 1664 deranged patients who were admitted into the Bethlehem Hospital in London, between the years 1784 and 1794, he tells us 910 of them were between the ages mentioned by Mr. Pinel. But the proportion of maniacal patients, above twenty and under fifty years of age, was much greater in the Pennsylvania Hospital in the month of April 1812. It was ascertained by Dr. Vandyke to be 68 out of 79, that is, nearly seven-eighths of their whole number. From the state of the body and mind within those periods, it is easy to account for this being the case. The blood-vessels and the nerves are then in a highly excitable state, and the former readily assume morbid or inflammatory action from the remote and exciting causes of disease. The mind too, within those years, possesses more sensibility, and of course is more easily acted upon by mental irritants, the sources of which from family afflictions, and disappointments in the pursuits of business, pleasure and ambition, are more numerous in those years, than in any of the previous or subsequent stages of life.

Madness, it has been said, seldom occurs under puberty. To the small number of instances of it that are upon record, I shall add four more. Two boys, the one of eleven, and the other of seven years of age, were admitted into our Hospital with this disease (the latter during the time of my attendance in 1799) and both discharged cured. I have since seen an instance of it in the year 1803, in a child of two years old, that had been affected with cholera infantum; and another in a child of the same age, in the year 1808, that was affected with internal dropsy of the brain. They both discovered the countenance of madness, and they both attempted to bite, first their mothers, and afterwards their own flesh. The reason why children and persons under puberty are so rarely affected with madness must be ascribed to mental impressions, which are its most frequent cause, being too transient in their effects, from the instability of their minds, to excite their brains into permanently diseased actions. It is true, children are often affected with delirium, but this is a symptom of general fever, which is always induced, like the few cases of madness in children that I have mentioned, only by corporeal causes.

From the records of the Bicetre Hospital, in France, it appears that madness rarely occurs in old age. Doleus and Dr. Greding mention several cases of it; the latter in a man of eighty-five. I have attended two men between sixty and seventy, and one woman between seventy and eighty, in the Pennsylvania Hospital, and a private patient in the eighty-first year of his age, in this disease. It has been said that maniacs seldom live to be old. I have known but few exceptions to this remark, and they were of persons in whom the extinction of the mind, in idiotism, had protected the body from being worn out prematurely by its constant and preternatural excitement or depression. One of the persons was Hannah Lewis, formerly mentioned, in whom the disease was induced by grief, in middle life, from the loss of her husband. She died in our Hospital in the year 1799, in the eighty-seventh year of her age. A predisposition to longevity, which she derived from her ancestors, predominated over the tendency of her long protracted disease to destroy her life. She lost one sister in the eighty-second year of her age, and at the time of her death had another living who was ninety-four, neither of whom had ever been affected with madness. There are two reasons why this disease so rarely attacks old people. Their blood vessels lose their vibratility from age, and hence they are less liable to fevers than in middle life; and from the diminution of sensibility in their nerves and brains, the causes of madness make but a feeble and transient impression upon their minds. In the latter condition of their bodies, they revert to that state which takes place in children, and which I have said protects them from the frequent occurrence of this disease.

V. Women, in consequence of the greater predisposition imparted to their bodies by menstruation, pregnancy, and parturition, and to their minds, by living so much alone in their families, are more predisposed to madness than men. A woman was admitted into our Hospital many years ago, who was deranged only during the time of her menstruation, and who in one of those periods hung herself with the string of her petticoat. Of 1664 patients admitted into the Bethlehem Hospital, between the years 1784 and 1794, eighty-four of them were women in whom madness followed parturition. I have been consulted in two cases, and I have heard of a third, in which madness was induced by the solitude of a country life, in women who had been accustomed to live in a large social and domestic society. Of 8874 patients admitted into the Bethlehem Hospital in London, between the years 1748 and 1794, four thousand eight hundred and thirty-two were women; nearly a fifth more than men. In St. Luke's Hospital in London, the proportion of women to men who have been admitted in a given number of years is in the ratio of three to two. But this disproportion of women to men who are affected with madness, is by no means universal. In a Hospital for mad people in Vienna, one hundred and seventeen men were admitted in a given number of years, and but ninety-four women. In a Hospital of the same kind at Berlin, twice as many males were admitted in a given time as females. More of the former than of the latter have been admitted into the Pennsylvania Hospital. In all these cases accidental circumstances, such as the want of accommodations suited to female delicacy, or deep rooted prejudices against public madhouses, and a preference of such as are private, may have lessened the proportion of women in the above instances, while the evils of war, bankruptcy, and habits of drinking, which affect men more than women, and which vary in their influence upon the mind in different countries, may have produced more instances of madness in the former than in the latter sex. Perhaps it would be correct to say, women are more subject to madness from natural causes, and men from such as are artificial.

What has been said under this head applies more particularly to general madness; but, from many facts, I am led to believe that men are more subject to that grade of derangement, which has been called hypochondriasm, than women. The distressing impressions made upon the minds of women frequently vent themselves in tears, or in hysterical commotions in the nervous system and bowels, while the same impressions upon minds of men pass by their more compact nervous and muscular fibres, and descend into the brain, and thus more frequently bring on hypochondriac insanity. If this remark be correct, it will confirm Dr. Heberden's assertion, that men are more disposed to suicide than women, for it necessarily follows their being most subject to that state of madness. Where the instances of suicide are more frequent among women than men, it is in those cases only in which the former are exposed to sudden paroxysms of vexation and despair.

VI. Single persons are more predisposed to madness than married people. Of seventy-two insane patients in the Pennsylvania Hospital, whose condition, relative to this question, was ascertained by my young friends Dr. Moore and Mr. Jenny, in the month of April 1812, forty-two had never been married, and five were widows and widowers, at the time they became deranged.

The absence of real and present care, which gives the mind leisure to look back upon past, and to anticipate future and imaginary evils, and the inverted operation of all the affections of the heart upon itself, together with the want of relief in conjugal sympathy from the inevitable distresses and vexations of life, and for which friendship is a cold and feeble substitute, are probably the reasons why madness occurs more frequently in single than in married people. Celibacy it has been said is a pleasant breakfast, a tolerable dinner, but a very bad supper. The last comparison will appear to be an appropriate one, when we consider further, that the supper is not only of a bad quality, but eaten alone. No wonder it sometimes becomes a predisposing cause of madness.

VII. The rich are more predisposed to madness than the poor, from their exposing a larger surface of sensibility to all its remote and exciting causes, Even where mental sensibility is the same in both those classes of people, the disease is prevented in the latter, by the constant pressure of bodily suffering, from labour, cold, and hunger. These present evils defend their minds from such as are past and anticipated; and these are the principal causes of madness. When it occurs in poor people, it is generally the effect of corporeal causes.

VIII. "Great wit, and madness," are said by Dryden "to be nearly allied." If he meant by this affinity between wit and madness, the rapid exercises of the mind in associating similar and dissimilar ideas or words which are peculiar to both, the remark is a correct one; but if he meant that great Wits are more predisposed to madness than other people, the remark is opposed by all that is known of the solidity of understanding, and correctness of conversation and conduct of Butler, Chesterfield, Franklin, Johnson, and many other distinguished men, who possessed the talent of wit in an eminent degree. Nor is the remark true if the term wit be intended to designate men of great understandings. Their minds are sometimes worn away by intense and protracted study, but they are rarely perverted by madness. The vigorous mind of Dean Swift perished gradually only from the former cause. Where madness has been induced by intense and protracted application to books, it has generally been in persons of weak intellects who were unable to comprehend the subjects of their studies.

IX. Certain occupations predispose to madness more than others. Pinel says, poets, painters, sculptors, and musicians, are most subject to it, and that he never knew an instance of it in a chemist, a naturalist, a mathematician, or a natural philosopher. The reason of this will be understood by recollecting what was said under the preceding head. The studies of the former exercise the imagination, and the passions, while the studies of the latter interest the understanding only. Dr. Arnold tells us, he has observed mechanics to be more affected with madness than merchants and members of the learned professions. This may arise from the vague and distracting exertions of genius, unassisted by education; or from corporeal causes, to which their employments expose them more than the classes of men that have been mentioned. Of the effects of the former of those causes, I once saw an instance in a house carpenter, who became deranged in consequence of an unsuccessful attempt to contrive a new kind of stair-case. More farmers it has been said become deranged than persons of the same grade of intellect and independence in cities. If this be the case, it must be ascribed to the greater solitude of their lives, more especially in the winter season, and to their being more exposed from labour and accidents, to its corporeal causes.

X. Certain climates predispose to madness. - It is very uncommon in such as are uniformly warm. Dr. Gordon informed me in his visit to Philadelphia in the year 1807, that he had never seen, nor heard of a single case of madness during a residence of six years in the province of Berbice. It is a rare disease in the West Indies. While great and constant heat increases the irritability of the muscles, it gradually lessens the sensibility of the nerves and mind, and the irritability of the blood-vessels, and in these I formerly supposed the predisposition to madness to be seated. It is more common in climates alternately warm and cold, but most so, in such as are generally moist and cold, and accompanied at the same time with a cloudy sky. Instances of it are said to be most frequent in England in the month of November, at which time the weather is unusually gloomy from the above causes. Even the transient occurrence of that kind of weather in the United States has had an influence upon this disease. In the month of May in the year 1806 it prevailed to a great degree, during which time three patients in the Pennsylvania Hospital made unsuccessful attempts upon their lives, and a fourth destroyed himself. Two instances of suicide occurred in the same month in Philadelphia.

XI. Certain states of society,, and certain opinions, pursuits, amusements, and forms of government, have a considerable influence in predisposing to derangement. It is a rare disease among savages. Baron Humboldt informed me, that he did not hear of a single instance of it among the uncivilized Indians in South America. Infidelity and atheism are frequent causes of it in Christian countries. In commercial countries, where large fortunes are suddenly acquired and lost, madness is a common disease. It is most prevalent at those times when speculation is substituted to regular commerce. The madhouses in England were crowded with patients before, and after the bursting of the South Sea bubble in the year 1720. In the United States, madness has encreased since the year 1790. This must be ascribed chiefly to an increase in the number and magnitude of the objects of ambition and avarice, and to the greater joy or distress, which is produced by gratification or disappointments in the pursuit of each of them. The funding system, and speculations in bank scrip, and new lands, have been fruitful sources of madness in our country. Sixteen persons perished from suicide in the city of New York, in the year 1804, in most of whom it was supposed to be the effect of madness, from the different and contrary events of speculation.

Even the profits and losses of regular trade and agricultural labour, now and then pervert the understanding. A respectable merchant died of madness in the Pennsylvania Hospital, in the year 1794, induced by a successful East India voyage. A farmer near Albany, who refused to take twenty shillings a bushel for a large quantity of wheat, in the year 1798 became insane from the sudden reduction of its price. Suicide was induced in a farmer of great wealth, in York county, in Pennsylvania, in the spring of 1812, by a similar disappointment, in obtaining a less price than he had been previously offered for a quantity of clover seed. Gaming is an occasional cause of madness in some countries. At Penang in the East Indies, where men often stake their wives upon the issue of a game, this disease is very common. The unfortunate gambler often rises from his seat in a fit of derangement, and sallies out into the street with instruments of murder in his hands. A bell is rung at this time, which drives people into their houses, to avoid being killed. A late German writer has remarked, that nervous diseases increase in the cities of Germany in proportion to the fondness of their citizens for seeing tragedies. It is easy to conceive they may extend their effects a little further, so as to excite morbid commotions in the blood-vessels of the brain. I have heard the greater frequency of madness in England, than in some other countries, ascribed in part to its inhabitants preferring tragedy to comedy, in their stage entertainments. The *real* emotions excited by these exhibitions of *imaginary* distress are never accompanied with an effort to relieve it, by which means there is an accumulation and reflux of sensation in the mind, that cannot fail of affecting the nerves and brain, and thereby to predispose to, or induce madness. Certain forms of government predispose to madness. They are those in which the people possess a just and exquisite sense of liberty, and of the evils of arbitrary power, against which complaints are stifled by a military force. The conflicting tides of the public passions, by their operation upon the understanding, become in these cases a cause of derangement. The assassination of tyrants and their instruments of oppression is generally the effect of this disease. That madness is thus induced, I infer from its occurring so rarely from a political cause in the United States. I have known but one instance of it, and that was in a gentleman who had been deranged some years before from debt, contracted by extravagant living. In a government in which all the power of a country is representative, and elective, a day of general suffrage, and free presses, serve, like chimnies in a house, to conduct from the individual and public mind, all the discontent, vexation, and resentment, which have been generated in the passions, by real or supposed evils, and thus to prevent the understanding being injured by them.

In despotic countries where the public passions are torpid, and where life and property are secured only by the extinction of the domestic affections, madness is a rare disease. Of the truth of this remark I have been satisfied by Mr. Stewart, the pedestrian traveller, who spent some time in Turkey: also by Dr. Scott, who accompanied lord M'Cartney in his embassy to China; and by Mr. Joseph Roxas, a native of Mexico, who passed nearly forty years of his life among the civilized but depressed natives of that country. Dr. Scott informed me that he heard of but a single instance of madness in China, and that was in a merchant who had suddenly lost 100,000l. sterling by an unsuccessful speculation in gold dust.

Mr. Carr, in his Northern Summer, tells us, that madness is an uncommon disease in Russia. It is a rare thing, says this professional traveller, to see a Russian peasant angry. He even persuades and reasons with his horse, when he wishes him to quicken his gait. It is to the long protracted civil and ecclesiastical tyranny of the late government of Spain, that we must ascribe the small number of maniacs in all the hospitals in that country. They amounted, according to Mr. Townsend, in the year 1786, to but 664, in a population which produces in Great Britain between 4,000 and 5,000; 2,600 of whom are in the city and neighbourhood of London. Habits of oppression in all those cases expend the excitability of the passions, and prevent their reacting upon the brain. But in some instances the understanding decays with the passions, in despotic countries. This state of the mind has been called fatuity. It is very common in Turkey and China. The inirritable or non-elastic state of the brain upon which this disorder depends, is induced in those countries without previous morbid excitement, in the same manner that the disorder called hepatalgia is induced, without previous hepatitis or obvious and sensible inflammation in the liver, in the East and West Indies.

XII. Revolutions in governments which are often accompanied with injustice, cruelty, and the loss of property and friends; and where this is not the case, with an inroad upon ancient and deep-seated principles and habits, frequently multiply instances of insanity. Mr. Volney informed me, in his visit to this city in the year 1799, that there were three times as many cases of madness in Paris in the year 1795, as there were before the commencement of the French Revolution. It was induced, I shall say hereafter, in several instances, by the events of the American Revolution.

XIII. Different religions, and different tenets of the same religion are more or less calculated to induce a predisposition to madness. Dr. Shebbeare says there are fewer instances of suicide (which is generally the effect of madness) in catholic, than in protestant countries. He ascribes it to the facility with which the Catholics relieve their minds from the pressure of guilt, by means of confession and absolution. This assertion and the reasoning founded upon it are rendered doubtful by 150 suicides having taken place in the catholic city of Paris in the year 1782, and but 32 in the same year in the protestant city of London. It is probable however the greater proportion of infidels in the former, than in the latter city at that time, may have occasioned the difference in the number of deaths in the two places, for suicide will naturally follow small degrees of insanity, where there are no habits of moral order from religion, and no belief in a future state. Dr. Shebbeare's assertion is rendered still less probable, by considering the usual effects of solitude upon the human mind, and this we know acts with peculiar force in the cells of monks and nuns. This remark is not the result of reasoning a priori. Of between 240 and 250 deranged people, who were confined at one time in a mad-house in the city of Mexico, Mr. Roxas informed me, in a great majority of them the disease had been contracted in those recluse and gloomy situations.

There are certain tenets held by several protestant sects of Christians which predispose the mind to derangement. They shall be noticed in another place.

I shall conclude the history of the remote exciting and predisposing causes of madness by the following remarks.

1. Its remote causes generally induce predisposing debility. Its exciting causes more commonly induce that morbid excitement in the blood-vessels of the brain in which madness is seated, but the sudden and violent action of a remote cause is often sufficient for that purpose without the aid of an existing cause.

2. Both the remote and exciting causes of madness produce their morbid effects more certainly, promptly, or slowly, according as the system is more or less predisposed to the disease by the causes formerly mentioned.

3. The predisposing causes of madness sometimes act with so much force, as to induce it without the perceptible co-operation of either a remote or an exciting cause. The remote causes of madness likewise act with so much force in some instances as to induce it without the perceptible cooperation of a predisposing or exciting cause.

Chapter Three - Of Partial Intellectual Derangement, and particularly of Hypochondriasis

Partial derangement consists in error in opinion, and conduct, upon some one subject only, with soundness of mind upon all, or nearly all other subjects. The error in this case is two-fold. It is directly contrary to truth, or it is disproportioned in its effects or expected consequences, to the causes which induce them. It has been divided by the nosologists according to its objects. When it relates to the persons, affairs, or condition of the patient only, and is attended with distress, it has been called hypochondriasis. When it extends to objects external to the patient, and is attended with pleasure, or the absence of distress, it has been called melancholia. They are different grades only, of the same morbid actions in the brain, and they now and then blend their symptoms with each other.

I wish I could substitute a better term than hypochondriasis, for the lowest grade of derangement. It is true the hypochondriac region is diseased in it; so it is after autumnal fevers, and yet we do not designate the obstructions induced by those fevers by that name. It would be equally proper to call every other form of madness hypochondriasis, for they are all attended with more or less disease or disorder in the liver, spleen, stomach and bowels, from which the name of hypochondriasis is derived. But I have another objection to that name, and that is, it has unfortunately been supposed to imply an imaginary disease only, and when given to the disease in question is always offensive to patients who are affected with it. It is true, it is seated in the mind; but it is as much the effect of corporeal causes as a pleurisy, or a bilious fever. Perhaps the term tristimania might be used to express this form of madness when erroneous opinions respecting a man's person, affairs, or condition, are the subjects of his distress.

I object likewise to the term melancholia, when used, as it is by Dr. Cullin, to express partial madness from external causes.

1. Because it is sometimes induced by causes that are not external to the patient, but connected with his person, affairs, or condition in life; and,

2. Because it conveys an idea of its being seated in the liver, and derived from vitiated or obstructed bile. Now the seat of the disease, from facts formerly mentioned, appears to be in the brain, and morbid or obstructed bile is evidently an accidental symptom of it. Perhaps it would be more proper to call it amenomania, from the errors that constitute it, being generally attended with pleasure, or the absence of distress.

The hypochondriasis, or tristimania, has sometimes been confounded with hysteria, but differs from it,

1. In being induced chiefly by mental causes, and particularly by such of them as act upon the understanding, through the medium of the passions and moral faculties. Hysteria is produced chiefly by corporeal causes. Its paroxysms only are excited by such as are mental. The chronic operation of the passions, so far from inducing it, sometimes cures it, or changes it into hypochondriasm.

2. In affecting men more than women.

3. In affecting chiefly persons of sedentary employments.

4. In the absence of globus hystericus.

5. In affecting the blood-vessels of the brain as well as the nerves. Hysteria affects the nerves and muscles only, and never the blood-vessels, so as to produce derangement, except for a short time, and only during its paroxysms.

6. The nerves in hypochondriasis are in a reverse state from that which takes place in hysteria. In the former, they are torpid, or in what Themison calls a *strictum* state. In the latter disease they are in a highly excitable, or what the same author has called a *laxum* state. These terms correspond with what Dr. Boerhaave has since denominated a *rigid* and *lax* state of the fibres.

7. Hypochondriasis is generally attended with costiveness or diarrhoea, and durable distress of mind, which are transient affections only in hysteria; and,

8. Hypochondriasis is relieved by warm weather, and warm drinks. Hysteria is made worse by each of them.

Hypochondriasis, or tristimania, is to hysteria what a typhus fever is to inflammatory fever. It is often combined with it, and sometimes alternates with it, and, when cured, it passes but of the system with symptoms of hysteria, in all those cases in which it was preceded by them. I beg the attention of the reader to this view of these two forms of disease. It is intended to destroy the nosological distinctions between them. As well might we divide the first and last stages of a fever by specific characters, as divide those two grades of morbid excitement by specific names.

I shall now deliver a history of the most characteristic symptoms of the two different forms of partial derangement that have been mentioned, and afterwards take notice of the remedies proper for each of them. I shall begin with *hypochondriasis* or *tristimania*.

The symptoms of this form of derangement as they appear in the body are, dyspepsia; costive ness or diarrhoea, with slimy stools; flatulency pervading the whole alimentary canal, and called in the bowels borborigmi; a tumid abdomen, especially on the right side; deficient or preternatural appetite; strong venereal desires, accompanied with nocturnal emissions of semen; or an absence of venereal desires, and sometimes impotence; insensibility to cold; pains in the limbs at times, resembling rheumatism; cough; cold feet; palpitation of the heart; headache; vertigo; tenitus aurium; a thumping like a hammer in the temples, and sometimes within the brain; a disposition to faint; wakefulness, or starting in sleep; indisposition to rise out of bed, and a disposition to lie in it for days, and even weeks; a cool and dry skin, and frequently of a sallow colour, from the want of a regular discharge of bile from the liver, and its absorption into the blood.

While the alimentary canal is thus depressed, and the blood-vessels, nerves and muscles, robbed of nearly all their excitement, or possess it in parts of the body only, the lymphatic system is often preternaturally excited; hence we frequently observe in this disease a constant and increased discharge of urine.

The characteristic symptom of this form of derangement, as it appears in the mind, is *distress,* the causes of which are numerous, and of a personal nature. I shall enumerate some of them, as they have appeared in different people. They relate, 1, to the patient's body. He erroneously believes himself to be afflicted with various diseases, particularly with consumption, cancer, stone, and above all, with impotence, and the venereal disease. Sometimes he supposes himself to be poisoned, or that his constitution has been ruined by mercury, or that the seeds of the hydrophobia are floating in his system.

2. He believes that he has a living animal in his body. A sea captain, formerly of this city, believed for many years that he had a wolf in his liver. Many persons have fancied they were gradually dying, from animals of other kinds preying upon different parts of their bodies. 3. He imagines himself to be converted into an animal of another species, such as a goose, a cock, a dog, a cat, a hare, a cow, and the like. In this case he adopts the noises and gestures of the animals into which he supposes himself to be transformed.

4. He believes he inherits, by transmigration, the soul of some fellow creature, but much oftener of a brute animal. There is now a madman in the Pennsylvania Hospital who believes that he was once a calf, and who mentions the name of the butcher that killed him, and the stall in the Philadelphia market on which his flesh was sold previously to his animating his present body.

5. He believes he has no soul. The late Dr. Percival communicated to me, many years ago, an account of a dissenting minister in England who believed that God had annihilated his soul as a punishment for his having killed a highway man by grasping him by the throat, who attempted to rob him. His mind was correct upon all other subjects.

6. He believes he is transformed into a plant. In the Memoirs of the Count de Maurepas we are told this error took possession of the mind of one of the princes of Bourbon to such a degree, that he often went and stood in his garden, where he insisted upon being watered in common with all the plants around him.

7. The patient afflicted with this disease sometimes fancies he is transformed into glass.

8. He believes, that by discharging the contents of his bladder, he shall drown the world.

9. He believes himself to be dead.

It is worthy of notice, in all these cases of erroneous judgment, the patients reason correctly, that is, draw just inferences from their errors. Thus the prince of Bourbon, when he supposed himself to be a plant, reasoned justly when he insisted upon being watered. In like manner, the hypochondriac who supposes himself to be dead, reasons with the same correctness when he stretches his body and limbs upon a bed, or a board, and assumes the stillness and silence of the shroud.

It is remarkable further, that all the erroneous opinions persons affected with this form of derangement entertain of themselves are of a degrading nature.

But again. The distress of a hypochondriac is derived from errors respecting, 1, his outward circumstances as they relate to his property.

2. The conduct of his friends, relations, or a mistress.

3. His birth place, and the society of his family, when absent from them.

4. The state of his country,

5. His spiritual state.

The mind, in its distress from all the above causes, is in a reverse state from that which was just now mentioned, in drawing erroneous, or disproportionate, conclusions from just premises. Thus the hypochondriac who possesses an income which he admits to be equal to all the exigencies of his family, reasons unjustly when he anticipates ending his days in a poor-house. In like manner the deranged penitent judges correctly when he believes that he has offended his Maker, but he reasons incorrectly when he supposes he has excluded him from his mercy.

In the hypochondriasis from all the causes that have been mentioned, the patients are for a while peevish and sometimes irascible. The lightest noises, such as the grating of a door upon its hinges, or its being opened and shut suddenly, produce in them anger or terror. They quarrel with their friends and relations. They change their physicians and remedies, and sometimes they discover the instability of their tempers by settling and unsettling themselves half a dozen times in different parts of their native country, or different foreign countries, in the course of a few years, leaving each of them with complaints of their climate, provisions, and the manners of their inhabitants.

The hypochondriasis, or tristimania, like most other diseases, has paroxysms, and remissions or intermissions, all of which are influenced by many circumstances, particularly by company, wine, exercise, and, above all, the weather.

A pleasant season, a line day, and even the morning sun, often suspend the disease. Mr. Cowper, who knew all its symptoms by sad experience, bears witness to the truth of this remark, in one of his letters to Mr. Haley. "I rise," says he, "cheerless and distressed, and brighten as the sun goes on." Its paroxysms are sometimes denominated "low spirits." They continue from a day, a week, a month, a season, to a year, and sometimes longer. The intervals differ, 1, in being accompanied with preternatural high spirits. 2, In being attended with remissions only; and, 3, with intermissions, or, in other words, with correctness and equanimity of mind.

The extremes of low and high spirits which occur in the same person, at different times, are happily illustrated by the following case. A physician in one of the cities of Italy was once consulted by a gentleman who was much distressed with a paroxysm of this intermitting state of hypochondriasm. He advised him to seek relief in convivial company, and recommended to him in particular to find out a gentleman of the name of Cardini, who kept all the tables in the city to which he was occasionally invited in a roar of laughter. "Alas! Sir," said the patient, with a heavy sigh, "I am that Cardini." Many such characters, alternately marked by high and low spirits, are to be found in all the cities in the world.

But there are sometimes flashes of apparent cheerfulness, and even of mirth, in the intervals of this disease, which are accompanied with latent depression of mind. This appears to have been the case in Mr. Cowper: hence, in one of his letters to Mr. Hayley, he says, "I am cheerful upon paper, but the most distressed of all creatures." It was probably in one of these opposite states of mind that he wrote his humorous ballad of John Gilpin.

In the history of hypochondriasm, as far as it has been given, there is a combination of some of the symptoms of hysteria from the nervous system being partially or alternately in a strictum or laxum, or, in other words, in an inirritable or irritable state, and from the blood-vessels being alternately in a diseased and sound state.

This mixture of the symptoms of hypochondriasis and hysteria, in those two opposite states of the system, is described with great accuracy in the following letter from a gentleman in Virginia, which I received a few years ago, containing the history of his own case.

Sir,

"I write to you to seek relief in a case of disease of the most inveterate, though not uncommon, nature. It is a nervous affection of the most obstinate kind. An apathy and torpor of the bowels and stomach, and a susceptibility of the mind exceeding all description: loss of sleep to an alarming degree at times, and the consequent debility, despair, subsultus tendinum, and paralytic sensations in many parts of my body, are the principal evils I suffer. My mind is liable to be excited by trifling and unsubstantial causes; disposed to cleave to unpleasant usages, to dwell on dreadful consequences from really trifling circumstances, to be appalled with vain apprehensions, and to cherish disgusts and disagreeable associations; indeed, to labour under a *fixidity* of ideas which causes my misery. I was attacked in the winter 1800 and 1801, and since that time have suffered an immensity of distress, with long intervals, however, of capacity for enjoyment. Moral causes are the sources of mv afflictions. The barriers of reason are cobwebs to oppose to the intrusion of this host of enemies. Am I in a convivial company? I think of some unpleasant circumstance. Do I eat heartily? I still think; my mind cannot rise above its customary state of feebleness. When I lie down, this fixed image presents itself. I am distressed, alarmed, my blood circulates rapidly, my brain is fired, a train of distressing ideas enter, and seize my mind: I am, as it were, all nerve; the least noise is like a shock of thunder, so that for seven years I have been in the constant habit of stopping both ears with wax; with intervals, however, of strength to bear noise, and sometimes even I am, as I think, almost well. I am within a few days of forty-four years of age; my appetite is always good; I eat every thing, drink moderately of wine, have found no good from any regimen, though I have not pursued any regimen but a very short time.

"I go to bed, my mind is distressed, I get a little quiet, and perhaps I am disposed to rest; at the moment of forgetfulness, which produces sound sleep, this image strikes my mind; I know what I am to suffer, am alarmed; my blood rushes through the jugular vessels; I hear my heart beat, and feel it thumping the whole night; my mind on fire, able to pursue no train of pleasant thought a moment; I get worse; despair; think of nothing but my wretched condition, till at last I lose several nights sleep; my pulse is low and threaded, and at last nature makes an effort and gradually restores me. Such is almost always my course.

"I can assure you that no cause of distress vexes my mind in which my conscience or my honour is implicated, or which would be even noticed by others. If I could indulge in religious duties and contemplations, to which my heart, my judgment, and natural disposition would lead me, it would, I really believe, cure me; but previous to my first attack, near eight years ago, in a previous state of debility and nervous affection, which pressed hard on my spirits, I wished to read on religious subjects, until all at once impious and profane ideas struck my mind: my soul recoiled, was shocked; I tried to banish them; nothing would do; not a moment were those ideas absent; at least they seized so fast, that I lost many nights and days sleep; and I was brought near the grave. I got better, and overcome, in some sort, this immoral influence; but shall never be able to indulge as I wish in religious duties. My heart often expands with enthusiasm, and then I taste of the joys of heaven. Now, Sir, can this dreadful state of mind be cured? Can I be made to possess less feeling, and more resolution to resist moral influences on the mind; to bear vexatious or distressing incidents; and to break this association, this *fixidity* of ideas?

"My feet, particularly my left foot, are always cold; and when I labour under great anxiety, both feet have, when warm in bed, a sensation as if they were asleep (as we say) which is very distressing. My whole left side is affected more than the other; the auditory nerve of my left ear is affected curiously, and unpleasantly, with sharp sounds, as if a body touched the nerve: I cannot well describe it.

"If I could be tranquil, I should be well. Whenever I can be moved by ambitious prospects, or entertain a desire for distinction, or any such passion, I am well. This is sometimes the case. When hopes or wishes of this sort take possession of my mind, they drive out other impressions; then I feel well. Active employment, if I could get in it, would cure me, but I know of none. When I feel well, I am uncommonly cheerful, playful, and happy.

"Now, Sir, I beg you, in consideration of suffering humanity, to take my case into your serious consideration, and extend to me the benefit of your advice."

In proportion as the hypochondriac disease advances, the symptoms of the hysteria, which are generally combined with it in its first stage, disappear, and all the systems in which the disease is seated acquire a uniformly torpid or irritable state. The remissions and intermissions which have been described, cease, and even the transient blaze of cheerfulness, which now and then escapes from a heart smothered with anguish, is seen no more. The distress now becomes constant. "Clouds return after every rain." Not a ray of comfort glimmers upon the soul in any of the prospects or retrospects of life. "All is now darkness without and within." These poignant words were once uttered by a patient of mine with peculiar emphasis, while labouring under this stage of the disease. Neither nature nor art now possess a single beauty, nor music or poetry a single charm. The two latter often give pain, and sometimes offence. In vain do love and friendship, and domestic affection, offer sympathy or relief to the mind in this awful situation. Even the consolations of religion are rejected, or heard with silence and indifference. Night no longer affords a respite from misery. It is passed in distracting wakefulness, or in dreams more terrible than waking thoughts; nor does the light of the sun chase away a single distressing idea. "I rise in the morning," says Mr. Cowper, in a letter to Mr. Haley, "like an infernal frog out of Acheron, covered with the ooze and mud of melancholy." No change of place is wished for that promises any alleviation of suffering. "Could I be translated to paradise," says the same elegant historian of his own sorrows, in a letter to Lady Hesketh, "unless I could leave my body behind me, my melancholy would cleave to me there."

But the last and worst stage of this form of derangement remains yet to be described. After it has completely put off all its hysterical symptoms, the patients fly for relief to such stimuli as act upon the body, in order to counteract the insupportable pressure of distress upon their minds. They take snuff, or chew tobacco. They eat voraciously, and drink wine and spirits, or take laudanum, in large quantities, when they are able to procure them. Sometimes the pain of a bodily disease suspends for a short time their mental distress. Mr. Boswell, in his life of Dr. Johnson, relates a story of a London tradesman, who, after making a large fortune, retired into the country to enjoy it. Here he became deranged with hypochondriasis, from the want of employment. His existence became finally a burden to him. At length he was afflicted with the stone. In a severe paroxysm of this disease, a friend sympathised with him. "No, no," said he, "don't pity me, for what I now feel is ease, compared with that torture of mind from which it relieves me." A woman in this city bore a child while she was afflicted with this disease. She declared, immediately afterwards, that she felt no more pain from parturition, than from a trifling fit of the colic. Where counteracting pains of the body are not induced by nature or accident, to relieve anguish of mind, patients often inflict them upon themselves. Walking barefooted over ground covered with frost and snow was resorted to by a clergyman of great worth in England for this purpose. Cardan, an eminent physician of the fifteenth century, made it a practice to bite his lips and one of his arms, also to whip his legs with rods, in order to ease the distress of his mind. Kempfer tells us that prisoners in Japan, who often became partially deranged from distress, used to divert their mental anguish by burning their bodies with moxa. The same decree of pain, and for the same purpose, is often inflicted upon the body, by cutting and mangling it in parts not intimately connected with life. But bodily pain, whether from an accidental disease, or inflicted by the patients upon themselves, is sometimes insufficient to predominate over the distress of their minds. Dr. Heberden mentions an instance of a man who was naturally so much afraid of pain that he dreaded even being bled, who in a fit of low spirits cut off his penis and scrotum with a razor, and declared, after he recovered the natural and healthy state of his mind, that he felt not the least pain from that severe operation. A similar instance of insensibility to bodily pain is related by Dr. Ruggieri, an Italian physician, of a hypochondriac madman of the name of Loval, who fixed himself upon a cross, and inflicted the same wounds upon himself, as far as he was able, that had been inflicted upon our Saviour. He was discovered in this situation, and taken down alive. During the paroxysms of his madness, he felt no pain from dressing his wounds, but complained as soon as they were touched, in the intervals of his disease. But this is not all. Hypochondriac distress seeks relief in an evil still greater than bodily pain. Can any thing be anticipated more dreadful than universal madness? and yet I once attended a lady in this city, whose sufferings from low spirits were of such a nature, that she ardently wished she might lose her reason, in order thereby to be relieved from the horror of her thoughts. This state of mind was not new in this disease. Shakespeare has described it in the following lines, in his inimitable history of all the forms of derangement, in the tragedy of King Lear. They are as truly philosophical, as they are poetical.

-------------- "Better I were distract;
So should my thoughts be sever'd from my griefs,
And woes, by wrong imaginations, lose
The knowledge of themselves."

But the most awful symptom of this disease remains yet to be mentioned, and that is despair. The marks of the extreme misery included in this word are sometimes to be seen in the countenances and gestures of hypochondriacs in a Hospital; but as it is difficult to obtain from such persons a history of their feelings, I shall endeavour to give some idea of them in the following account, communicated to me by a clergyman who passed four years and a half in that state of mind.

He said "he felt the bodily pains and mental anguish of the damned; that he slumbered only, but never slept soundly, during the long period that has been mentioned; that he lost his appetites? and passions, so as to desire and relish nothing, and to love and hate no one; that his feet were constantly cold, and the upper part of his body warm; that he lost all sense of years, months, weeks, days, and nights, and even of morning and evening; that in this respect, time was to him, no more." During the whole period of his misery, he kept his hands in constant motion towards his head and thighs, and ceased not constantly to cry out, "wretched man that I am! I am damned; oh, I am damned everlastingly."

Terrible as this picture of despair is, the disease has symptoms which mark a still greater degree of misery. It sometimes creates such a disgust of life, as to make the subjects of it wish to die. How undescribable, and even incomprehensible, must be that state of mind, which thus extinguishes the deep seated principle of the love of life! In the exquisite tortures of the stone, and colic, and even under the progress of an excruciating and mortal cancer, men are willing, nay anxious, to live; of course the sufferings from the anguish of mind I have described, exceed the sufferings from those diseases. But there is a symptom of despair which places its horrors beyond a mere *wish to die*. It often drives the distracted subject of it to precipitate the slow approaches of death with his own hand. A pistol, a razor, a river, a mill-dam, a halter, or laudanum, are the means usually resorted to for this purpose. Sometimes the instruments of death are of a more painful nature. I have once seen the body of a Russian officer mangled with thirteen wounds inflicted' by himself. He had fallen into despair in consequence of debts contracted in a foreign country. Sometimes a horror is entertained by persons in this situation at the crime of suicide, but, in order to escape from life, they provoke death from the hands of government by committing murder; many instances of this kind are to be met with, not only in the records of medicine, but in our public newspapers. Dreadful as this state of mind is, there is one still more distressing, and that is the desire, and fear of death operating alternately upon the mind. I have seen this state of hypochondriasm. It was in the lady who wished to be relieved from the horror of her thoughts by the complete loss of her reason.

After the history that has been given of the distress, despair, and voluntary death, which are induced by that partial derangement which has been described, I should lay down my pen, and bedew my paper with my tears, did I not know that the science of medicine has furnished a remedy for it, and that hundreds are now alive, and happy, who were once afflicted with it. Blessed science! which thus extends its friendly empire, not only over the evils of the bodies, but over those of the minds, 'of the children of men!

Chapter Four - Of the Remedies for Hypochondriasis or Tristimania

The remedies for this form of derangement divide themselves into two classes.

I. Such as are intended to act directly upon the body; and,

II. Such as are intended to act indirectly upon the body, through the medium of the mind.

1. Before we proceed to administer the remedies that are indicated under our first head, it will be proper carefully to review the history of all the remote and exciting causes of this disease, and, when possible, to remove them. If this be impracticable, or if the disease continue from habit after all its causes have been removed, recourse should be had to,

1. **Bloodletting,** if the pulse be tense, or full; or depressed, without either fulness, or tension. I have prescribed this remedy with success, and thereby in several instances suddenly prepared the way for its being cured in a few days by other medicines. I was led to use it by the following fact, communicated to me by the late Dr. Thomas Bond. A preacher among the Friends called upon him, to consult him in this state of madness. He said he was possessed of a devil, and that he felt him constantly in aches and pains in every part of his body. The Doctor felt his pulse, which he found to be full and tense. He advised him to sit-down in his parlour, and persuaded him to let him open a vein in his arm. While the blood was flowing the patient cried out, "I am relieved, I felt the devil fly out of the orifice in my vein as soon as it was opened." From this time he recovered rapidly from his derangement. The

advantages of bleeding are evinced still further by the relief obtained in this disease by the loss of blood from the hemorrhoidal vessels, and by other accidental haemorrhages. But, if experience had not thus established the efficacy of this remedy, its use would be suggested by the habits of such patients, of indulging their appetites, not only to satisfy hunger, but to suspend their distress; and by congestions of blood in the liver and spleen, which usually take place in this disease. After bleeding, if it be required,

2. **Purges** should be given. They are indicated by the obstructions of the viscera, and torpor of the alimentary canal. They often bring away black bile, and sometimes worms. The more active purges, particularly aloes, jalap, and calomel, should be preferred in this disease. The daughters of Prcetus, who supposed themselves to be cows, were cured by Melampus by means of hellebore, which is of a purging nature. The medicine has ever since bore his name.

3. **Emetics,** by exciting the stomach, often remove morbid excitement from the brain, and thus restore the mind to its healthy state. They moreover assist purges in exciting the alimentary canal, and in dislodging obstructions from the abdominal viscera.

4. **A reduced diet,** consisting of food and drinks that contain but little nourishment should be combined with the three remedies that have been mentioned. As the stomach is frequently in a dyspeptic state, the aliment and drinks should consist of such articles as are least disposed to increase or produce a morbid acid in it.

After reducing the action of the blood-vessels to a par of debility with the nervous system, or, to borrow an allusion from a mechanical art, after *plumbing* those two systems, the remedies should consist,

5. **Of Stimulating Aliment, drinks and medicines**.

The *diet* should consist of solid animal food, with such vegetables as are least disposed to acidity, and both should be rendered palatable by condiments. The *drinks* should consist of old Madeira or sherry wine, and porter diluted with water, or taken alone, provided the stomach be not affected with a morbid acid, I have once known this disease cured by the liberal use of Madeira wine. In some cases, old claret is better received by the stomach than the white wines, from its containing less fermentable matter in it. The drinks should be taken warm, for the stomach is generally too weak to react under the sedative operation of such as are cold. Warm tea and coffee, made weak, are generally grateful to the stomach, and should be advised, when it is not affected with dyspepsia. The celebrated Mr. Burke often relieved the low spirits which were induced by the solicitude and vexations of his political life, by sipping a tea-cup full of hot water. In cases of dyspepsia, or indigestion, as little drink as possible should be taken with food. The *medicines* proper in this disease should be the different preparations of iron. I know they have been said to be hurtful in it. It is true they are often ineffectual, but this is because the system is reduced *below* their stimulus in their ordinary doses. When given in large doses, mixed with ginger, or black pepper, and the common bitters of the shops, and persisted in for several months, they are powerful medicines. Tar, in the form of pills, or infused in water, and garlic in substance, or infused in peppermint tea, afford great relief in this disease, more especially when the stomach is affected. Magnesia, lime-water and milk, and the alkaline salts, should be given to relieve acidity in the stomach, should that symptom of dyspepsia call for them. Assafoetida is an excellent medicine in this depressed state of the system, and preferable to any of the common foetid gums that are in use to exhilarate the spirits. But our principal reliance for this purpose should be upon opium. Mr. Cowper says, ten drops of laudanum, taken occasionally, saved him from being "devoured by melancholy." This noble medicine, which has been happily called "the medicine of the mind," has many advantages over ardent spirits as a cordial. It affords more prompt relief; and a habit of attachment to it is more slowly formed, and more easily broken. It does not pollute the breath, nor does it ever tend to excite, or increase that hysterical irritability of temper which is sometimes connected with this disease. However useful ardent spirits may be in transient diseases, they cannot be used in such as are of a chronic nature, without inducing such a fondness for them as not only to prevent their acting as remedies, but to convert them into poisons, often alike fatal to the soul and body.

6. **The warm bath,** applied in the form of water, or vapour, and rendered more stimulating, if necessary, by the addition of saline or aromatic substances to it. The heat of the water should be a little above that of the body. It does most service when it induces sweats. Mr. Cowper was always relieved by that discharge from his skin.

7. **The cold bath.** This remedy should not be advised until the system has been prepared for it by the previous use of the warm bath.

8. **Frictions** to the trunk of the body and limbs. These tend very much to excite the cutaneous extremities of the nerves and blood-vessels, and thus to equalize the excitement of the system. I have known two instances in which a recovery from this disease succeeded an attack of the itch. - The remedy in this case was probably the pleasurable sensation excited by scratching, in order to relieve it.

9. **Exercise,** especially upon horseback. *Labour* is still more useful, particularly in the open air.

10. **The excitement of pain**. I mentioned the accidental effects of the pain of a stone in the bladder, and of burning moxa on the body, in suspending anguish of mind in the history of this disease. It may be excited in various ways. Mustard to the feet is generally sufficient for this purpose. I once attended a gentleman from Barbadoes, who suffered great distress of mind from a hypochondriac gout which floated in his nerves and brain; but no

sooner did the gout fix, and excite pain in his hands or feet, than he recovered his spirits, and became pleasant and agreeable to all around him.

11. **Salivation.** Mercury acts in this disease, 1, by abstracting morbid excitement from the brain to the mouth. 2, By removing visceral obstructions. And, 3, by changing the cause of our patient's complaints, and fixing them wholly upon his sore mouth. The salivation will do still more service if it excite some degree of resentment against the patient's physician or friends. - The effects of mercury in this disease, have sometimes been compared to those of a handful of shot shaken in a bottle, lined with filth and dirt, in order to clean it. It stimulates every part of the body, renders the vessels pervious to their natural juices, conveys morbid action out of the body by the mouth, and thus restores the mind to its native seat in the brain,

12. **Blisters and issues** have been found useful in this form of madness. They are calculated to excite the action of the skin, and to produce what has been happily called a centrifugal direction of the fluids. They are more particularly indicated, if the disease have been induced by eruptions repelled from the skin.

II. We come next in order to mention the remedies for the body, which are intended to act through the medium of the mind. The first thing to be done by a physician, under this head, is to treat the disease in a serious manner. To consider it in any other light, is to renounce all observation in medicine. However erroneous a patient's opinion of his case may be, his disease is a *real* one. It will be necessary, therefore, for a physician to listen with attention to his tedious and uninteresting details of its symptoms and causes. In some cases, patients wish to think their diseases are trifling, and attended with no danger, but in hypochondriasis, they are always best satisfied in believing their disease to be difficult and dangerous. A physician should carefully avoid likewise speaking lightly of his patient's disease to his friends and neighbours, for he will take uncommon pains to discover, from them, his opinion of his case, and if it be different from that which has been given to him, he will not only reproach him with a want of candour, but will immediately seek relief from another physician. I once knew an instance of this kind in this city. The patient refused to see the physician afterwards, who had thus deceived him. In the worst grade of this disease, he will not bear contradiction, and hence it will be necessary to conform our remedies as much as possible to his erroneous opinions of the nature of his disease. If he believe himself to be affected with any of the diseases that were formerly named, medicines must be prescribed for them, and administered in a manner calculated to act upon his principle of faith, and to beget his confidence in them. In the more moderate grade of his errors upon the subject of his disease, contradiction, and reasoning, may be opposed to them. When these means are employed, the conduct of a physician should correspond with them. I once injured myself, and my patient, who supposed himself to be affected with the venereal disease, by prescribing for him a few mercurial pills, in compliance with his earnest solicitations, after having assured him that he had not a particle of its virus in his system. I have in several instances removed all doubt upon the subject, by advising matrimony, or a renewal of conjugal intercourse, if my patients were married, and by offering; them at the same time a bond for a large sum of money, if any bad consequences should follow their obedience to my advice. In this way I have made many gentlemen happy, and never in a single instance incurred the least discredit or blame.

Persons afflicted with this form of derangement, I said formerly, now and then believe themselves to be poisoned. In this case it is sometimes necessary to humour their error, and to prescribe suitable means to remove it. Dr. Cox, in his Treatise upon Insanity, has furnished us with an excellent precedent for this purpose. A gentleman in England supposed a shirt which he had worn had been poisoned by his maid, and determined to subject her to the punishment of the law. His physician humoured his belief and resentment, by pretending to have discovered a poisonous matter in his shirt, by means of some chemical experiments upon it, and concurred with him in prosecuting his maid for an intended murder. A new course was hereby given to his thoughts, and a new action excited in his brain, by which he was perfectly cured.

Terror once cured, for a while, a patient of mine, of a belief that he had been poisoned by taking arsenic as a medicine, and that it had eaten out his bowels. A student of medicine, to whom he told this tale, attempted to convince him of his error, upon which he begged him to open him, and to satisfy himself by examining the cavity of his belly. After some preparation, the student laid him upon a table, and drew the back of a knife from one extremity of his belly to the other. "Stop, stop," said my patient, "I've got guts," and suddenly escaped from the hands of his operator. His cure would probably have been durable, after the use of this remedy, had not real distress from another cause brought back that which was imaginary.

If our patient imagine he has a living animal in his body, and he cannot be reasoned out of a belief of it, medicines must be given to destroy it; and if an animal, such as he supposes to be in his body, should be secretly conveyed into his close stool, the deception would be a justifiable one, if it served to cure him of his disease.

If our patient should believe himself to be transformed into an animal of another species by transmigration, or in any other way, our remedies should be accommodated to the grade of his madness, and the nature of the animal into which he supposes himself to be changed. Ridicule has sometimes been employed with success in such cases. Mr. Pinel mentions an instance of its sudden efficacy in curing a watch-maker in Paris, who believed that his head had been cut off, and that he carried the head of a man who had been guillotined, instead of his own.

A physician, formerly of this city, used to divert his friends, by relating the history of a cure which had been performed of a patient in this form of madness, who believed himself to be a plant. One of his companions, who favoured his delusion, persuaded him he could not thrive without being watered, and while he made the patient believe, for some time, he was pouring water from the spout of a tea-pot, discharged his urine upon his head. The remedy in this case was resentment and mortification.

Cures of patients, who suppose themselves to be glass, may easily be performed by pulling a chair, upon which they are about to sit, from under them, and afterwards showing them a large collection of pieces of glass as the fragments of their bodies.

An unwillingness to discharge the contents of the bladder, from the cause that has been mentioned, was once cured by persuading the patient that the world was on fire, and that nothing but his water would extinguish it. This error was cured by Dr. Ferriar by means of an emetic, which, by its action upon the stomach, destroyed the command of the patient's will over the sphincter of the bladder.

I have heard of a person afflicted with this disease, who supposed himself to be dead, who was instantly cured by a physician proposing to his friends, in his hearing, to open his body, in order to discover the cause of his death.

In all the cases that have been mentioned, of error and distress which relate to the body only, similar advantages would probably arise from exciting fear or anger, or any other powerful emotion of the mind.

I attended a young man in the year 1806, who cherished an obstinate hypochondriac belief, after his recovery from the autumnal fever, that he should die, and felt at the same time a great dread of death. I assured him over and over that he was in no danger, but without being able to inspire him with the least expectation of life. In one of my visits to him, I asked him, upon entering his room, how he was; "very bad," said he, and repeated his belief that he should soon die. - His nurse, who sat by him, added, that he had fixed upon an hour in the approaching night as the time for his dissolution. After pausing a few moments, I asked him if I should send a joiner to measure him for his coffin. This question instantly gave a new current to his feelings, and from that time he recovered rapidly; nor did he ever mention an apprehension of dying to me, in any of my subsequent visits to him. Anger had uniformly the same beneficial effects upon a gentleman in Maryland, who, when in health, was accustomed to speculate upon controverted subjects in religion. There was an opinion held by one sect of Christians, which he held in great abhorrence. His friends, who knew this, always contrived, when they saw him unusually dejected, to provoke a controversy with him upon the subject that was hateful to him. It never failed to rouse his resentment, and thereby to banish, for a while, a paroxysm of his disease.

If debt be the cause of our patient's disease, we may presume it has been incurred with a clear conscience, and a fair character, for a dishonest man seldom feels distress enough from this cause to bring on disease. In this case we must advise our patient to take the benefit of our insolvent and bankrupt laws. Many men have been thus saved from a miserable death, and restored to health, and usefulness to their families and society.

If the disease has been induced by the supposed or real ingratitude, neglect, or ill usage of friends or relations, there are two modes of treating it; one consists in advising forgiveness, of contempt of the injury; the other, in exciting a moderate degree of anger against the persons who have offended or injured our patients. This anger, by its stimulus, counteracts the depression both of the body and mind. It should be carefully guarded from venting itself in acts of malice or revenge.

If the disease be induced by nostalgia, or what is called home-sickness, the patient should be advised to visit his native country. It was once cured by this means in a Welsh soldier in the British army. When this remedy cannot be employed, it should be opposed, by exciting a powerful or active counter passion. In the year 1733 general Praxin led a Russian army to the banks of the Rhine. At this remote distance from their native country, five or six soldiers became unfit for duty every day from home sickness. The general issued an order to bury alive all who were affected with it. This punishment was inflicted in two or three instances, in consequence of which the disease instantly disappeared from the army. Fear, excited by a far less cruel remedy, I have no doubt would have had the same effect.

The remedies for this disease, when brought on by disappointed love, and by grief, shall be mentioned, when we come to treat of the cure of the diseases of the passions.

It will naturally occur to the reader that the three last causes of hypochondriac madness will be concealed by a patient from the knowledge of a physician. But they must be extorted, by direct or indirect means, or the appropriate remedies cannot be employed to remove their hurtful influence upon the system.

If the derangement of our patient has been induced by the real or supposed distresses of his country, it will be proper to advise him to avoid reading news-papers, and conversing upon political subjects, and thereby to acquire a total ignorance of public events. But if he object to this remedy, he should be advised to take a part in the disputes which divide his fellow citizens. In favour of this conduct, I shall mention a single fact. There was a form of this disease, well known during the revolutionary war in several of the states by the names of the tory rot, and the protection fever. It was confined exclusively to those friends of Great Britain, and to those timid Americans, who took no public part in the war. Many of them died of it, but not a single whig nor royalist, who took an active part in the revolution, was affected with it. This was the more remarkable, as many of them lost their fortunes and former rank in society, by their exertions in support of the principles and measures to which they had devoted their passions or their lives. By eating garlic, we become insensible of the breath of persons that has been rendered offensive by it. In like manner, by imbibing a portion of party spirit, we become insensible of the vices and follies of our associates in politics, and thus diminish more or less than one half (according to the number of our party) this source of hypochondriacal derangement. Happily for our citizens, the disease that has been named has passed away with the events of the American revolution, and from the general operation of the above remedies, as well as from causes formerly mentioned, it has rarely been succeeded by any other form of political hypochondriasm in the United States.

If the disease be derived from a sense of guilt, it is generally connected with ignorance, or erroneous opinions in religion. The former must be removed, by advising the visits of a sensible and enlightened clergyman. The latter consist, generally in our patient's believing one or both the following errors: 1. That he is excluded from the divine mercy by an irreversible decree of the Supreme Being, or, in other words, that he was created on purpose to be made miserable for ever. - The second error believed by our patient is, that he has committed the unpardonable sin. To the first error we may reply, that there is no pagan opinion more contrary to nature and reason, and to the whole tenor, as well as to the most consistent interpretations, of the Scriptures, than the doctrine of men being called into existence on purpose to endure the pains of eternal misery. To the second error we may reply, that no two divines agree in what constitutes the unpardonable sin; that many wise and good men believe it is not possible to commit it, in the present state of the gospel dispensation, and all divines agree that "no man had committed it, who was afraid he had." It is of consequence to a physician, to be fully prepared upon the subjects of the two errors that I have named, for they are the two principal causes of religious hypochondriasm.

In the application of all these remedies to the mind, it is of consequence to know that there are acquiescing, reasoning, contradicting, and ridiculing points in this disease, *above* which they respectively do harm, and *below* which they are of no efficacy.

In all cases it will be proper to seduce patients from conversing upon their disease. "Conversation upon melancholy," says Dr. Johnson, "feeds it;" for which reason he advises his friend Boswell, who was subject to it, "never to speak of it, to his friends, nor in company."

There are several other remedies which act upon the body through the medium of the mind, and that are proper, in this disease from all its causes. The first of these is, the **destruction** of all old associations of ideas. Every thing a hypochondriac patient sees or hears, becomes tinctured with some sad idea of his disease. Hence the same objects and sounds never fail of renewing the remembrance of it. Change therefore his dress, his room, his habitation, and his company, as often as possible. A gentleman in South Carolina used to cure himself of a fit of low spirits by changing his clothes. Even change his person as much as possible. Long nails, a long beard, and uncombed hair, often become exciting causes of a paroxysm of this disease. They should therefore be carefully prevented or removed.

2. **Employment,** or business of some kind. Man was made to be active. Even in paradise he was employed in the healthy and pleasant exercises of cultivating a garden. Happiness, consisting in folded arms, and in pensive contemplation, beneath rural shades, and by the side of purling brooks, never had any existence, except in the brains of mad poets, and love-sick girls and boys. Hypochondriac derangement has always kept pace with the inactivity of body and mind which follows wealth and independence in all countries. It is frequently induced by this cause in those citizens, who retire, after a busy life, into the country, without carrying with them a relish for agriculture, gardening, books, or literary society.

Building, commerce, a public employment, an executorship to a will; above all, agriculture, have often cured this disease. The last, that is, agriculture, by agitating the passions by alternate hope, fear, and enjoyment, and by rendering bodily exercise or labour necessary, is calculated to produce the greatest benefit. Great care should however be taken, never to advise retirement to a part of the country where good society cannot be enjoyed upon easy terms.

In those cases in which the body cannot be employed, the mind should be kept constantly busy. - Mr. Cowper often relieved his melancholy by reading novels. Hence he has well said,

> "*Absence* of occupation is not rest.
> A mind quite *vacant* is a mind *distrest.*"

I knew a lady in whom this disease was brought on by a disappointment in love, who cured herself by translating Telemachus into English verse. The remedy here was, chiefly, *constant* employment.

Dr. Burton, in his Anatomy of Melancholy, delivers the following direction for its cure: "Be not idle; be not solitary." Dr. Johnson has improved this advice by the following commentary upon it. "When you are idle, be not solitary; and when you are solitary, be not idle." The illustrious Spinola, upon hearing of the death of a friend, inquired of what disease he died? "Of having nothing to do," said the person who mentioned it. "Enough," said Spinola, "to kill a general." Not only the want of employment, but the want of care, often increases, as well as brings on this disease. This was exemplified in the two instances, formerly mentioned, of suicide being induced by situations in which the heart wished and cared for nothing.

Concerts, evening parties, and the society of the ladies, to gentlemen affected with this disease, have been useful. Of the efficacy of the last, Mr. Green has happily said,

> "With speech so sweet, so sweet a mien,
> They excommunicate the spleen."

3. Certain amusements. Those should be preferred, which, while they interest the mind, afford exercise to the body. The chase, shooting, playing at quoits, are all useful for this purpose. The words of the poet, Mr. Green, upon this subject, deserve to be committed to memory by all physicians.

> "To cure the mind's wrong bias, *spleen,*
> Some recommend the bowling green.
> Some hilly walks — *all*, exercise,
> *Fling but a stone* — the giant dies."

Chess, checkers, cards, and even push-pin, should be preferred to idleness, when the weather forbids exercise in the open air. The theatre has often been resorted to, to remove fits of low spirits; and it is a singular fact, that a tragedy oftener dissipates them than a comedy. The remedy, though distressing to persons with healthy minds, is like the temperature of cold water to persons benumbed with frost; it is exactly proportioned to the excitability of their minds, and it not only abstracts their attention from themselves, but even revives their spirits.

A female patient of mine, in whom this disease had several times been excited by family afflictions, lost a favourite child in November 1811, which produced many of its symptoms. Soon afterwards her husband became sick. The lighter and dissimilar distress occasioned by this event suddenly removed her disease, and she regained, with the recovery of her husband, her usual health and spirits. Mirth, or even cheerfulness, when employed as remedies in low spirits, are like hot water to a frozen limb. They are disproportioned to the excitability of the mind, and, instead of elevating, never fail to increase its depression, or to irritate it. Mr. Cowper could not bear to hear his humorous story of John Gilpin read to him in his paroxysms of this disease. It was to his "heavy heart," what Solomon happily compares to the conflict produced by pouring vinegar upon nitre, or in other words, upon an alkaline salt.

Certain objects, distinguished for their beauty or grandeur, often afford relief in this disease. Mr. Cowper experienced a transient elevation of spirits, from contemplating the ocean from the house of his friend Mr. Haley; and the unfortunate Mrs. Robinson soothed the gloom of her mind, by viewing the dashing of the waves of the same sublime object, by the light of the moon, at Brighton. Certain animals suspend the anguish of mind of this disease by their innocence, ingenuity or sports. Mr. Cowper sometimes found relief in playing with three tame hares, and in observing a number of leeches to rise and fall in a glass with the changes in the weather. The poet says,

> "*Laugh* and be *well*. Monkeys have been
> Extreme good doctors for the spleen.
> And kitten — if the humour hit,
> Has harlequin'd away the fit."

The famous Luther was cheered under his fits of low spirits by listening to the prattle, and observing the sports and innocent countenances of young children. The tone of their voices is probably a source of a part of the relief derived from their company. Mr. Cowper was always exhilarated by conversing with Mr. Hay ley's son, only because he was pleased with the soft and musical tones of his voice.

4. Music has often afforded great relief in this disease. Luther, who was sorely afflicted with it, has left the following testimony in its favour. "Next to Theology, I give the highest place to music, for thereby all anger is forgotten; the devil, also melancholy, and many tribulations and evil thoughts are driven away." For the same reason that tragedies afford more relief than comedies, plaintive tunes are more useful than such as are of a sprightly nature. I attend a citizen of Philadelphia, occasionally, in paroxysms of this disease, who informed me that he was cured of one of them by hearing the old hundred psalm tune sung in a country church. His disease, he said, instantly went off in a stream of tears. Dr. Cardan always felt a suspension of the anguish of his mind from the same cause; and Mr. Cowper tells his friend Mr. Hayley, in one of his letters, that he was "relieved as soon as his troubles gushed from his eyes." The tears in these cases acted by indirectly depleting from the brain.

It is remarkable, that sprightly tunes are as offensive as comic representations in this disease. This was once exemplified by a Mr. Derberow, formerly a patient in the Pennsylvania Hospital. In a fit of low spirits, he heard the sound of a lively tune from a flute in an adjoining room. He suddenly rushed into it, snatched the flute from the gentleman's hands who was playing upon it, and broke it in pieces upon his head.

5. Committing entertaining passages of prose and verse to **memory,** and copying manuscripts, have been found useful in relieving hypochondriasm. They divert and translate attention and action from the understanding to a sound part of the mind. Reading aloud has nearly the same effect.

6. Dr. Burton recommends, in the highest terms, the reading of the **bible** to hypochondriac patients. He compares it to an apothecary's shop, in which is contained remedies for every disease of the body. I have frequently observed the languor and depression of mind which occur in the evening of life, to be much relieved by the variety of incidents, and the sublime and comfortable passages, that are contained in that only true history of the origin, nature, duties, and future destiny of man. A captain Woodward, of Boston, who lately suffered all the hardships of shipwreck on an inhospitable island in the East Indies, found great comfort in revolving the history of Joseph and his brethren in his mind. A captain Inglefield revived his spirits, and those of his crew, in a similar situation, by telling them pleasant stories.

The mind requires a succession of connected events to divert it from itself, and this is the reason why stories of all kinds, which require constant attention to comprehend them, are so useful in this disease.

Where there is no relish for the simple and interesting stories contained in the Bible, the reading of novels should be recommended to our patients. They contain a series of supposed events which arrest the attention, and cause the mind to forget itself. It is because they so uniformly produce this effect that they are often resorted to by old people even of elevated understandings, in order to divert themselves from the depression of spirits which the death or treachery of friends, bodily pain, and the dread of futurity, create in their minds.

7. **Mentioning the name** of a parent, relation or friend, from whom the patient has received acts of kindness, protection, or relief, in early life. We fly from habit to those persons, when in distress in any part of our lives, who have succoured us under the pains and distresses of childhood. These persons are generally our parents. I once assisted in performing the operation of lithotomy upon a young gentleman in this city, whose only cry during the operation was, "O! my father, my father!" I have heard a woman utter the name of her mother only, during the whole time of the excision of a cancerous breast. I attended a young gentleman in our hospital in the year 1803 in this disease, who had lived with a most indulgent grandfather when a boy. In the lowest stage of his depression, the mentioning the name only, of his grandfather revived him, and often drew him into pleasant conversation. The same advantages might probably be derived, from carrying a patient's memory and imagination back to the innocent and delightful sports and studies of early life.

8. **Matrimony,** if our patients are single. The constant pursuits and wholesome cares of a family generally prevent and cure such as are transient and imaginary.

9. **Terror,** by the concussion it gives to both body and mind, has sometimes cured this disease. A lady in New York, in whom it was induced by the habitual use of opium, was cured by this remedy, administered by the hand of her physician. In one of his visits to her, he took a large snuffbox out of his pocket. She looked at it as if she wished for a pinch of snuff. The physician put it into her hands. Upon opening it, an artificial snake that had been coiled up in it, suddenly leaped upon her shoulder. She was convulsed with terror, and from time left off the use of opium, and rapidly recovered. She lived forty years afterwards in good health, and finally died about eighty years of age.

10. **Travelling.** Long journeys should be preferred to short excursions from home. They relieve the mind from a monotony of objects, and awaken a constant succession of new ideas. They moreover create a necessity for constant bodily exertion, and they remove the patient from the society of his friends, who, by being obliged to listen to his complaints, add fuel to his disease.

The journeys in those cases should be to a warm climate, and the patient should be advised, before he leaves home, to change every article of his dress, even the furniture of his pockets, that he may see nothing while abroad, that can revive his disease by association.

In the history of this disease I remarked that there is in hypochondriacs a disposition to inflict pain upon their bodies by means of wounds, in order to suspend anguish of mind. This should be prevented by removing all the instruments out of their way that are usually employed for that purpose. Sometimes this anguish of mind, I have said, leads its miserable subjects to seek to put an end to their existence by their own hands. This should be prevented, not only by depriving them of all the means of destroying themselves, but by securing the windows and doors in which they are confined, and never permitting them to be alone; also by such other means as accident or design have proved to be successful, and which act upon the mind through the medium of the body, and upon the body through the medium of the mind. These are wine, blood-letting, an unexpected sense of pain, compassion, a sudden and violent exertion of the active powers of the body and mind, terror, a sense of shame, and, lastly, infamy. I shall briefly mention instances of the efficacy of each of them in preventing suicide.

1. A gentleman afflicted with this disease went with a loaded pistol into a tavern in London, with a design to destroy himself. To conceal his intention, he called for a small decanter of wine, and, after locking the door of the room into which he had been conducted, cocked his pistol, but before he discharged its contents through his head, determined to try the quality of his wine. Perceiving it to be very good, he drank a second, and then a third glass, after which he uncocked his pistol, and finished the whole decanter. Finding such a prompt remedy for his despair in this cordial liquor, he continued to use it freely, and was thereby cured.

2. In the year 1803 I visited a young gentleman in our hospital, who became deranged from remorse of conscience in consequence of killing a friend in a duel. His only cry was for a pistol, that he might put an end to his life. I told him, the firing of a pistol would disturb the patients in the neighbouring cells, and that the wound made by it would probably cover his cell with blood, but that I could take away his life in a more easy and delicate way, by bleeding him to death, from a vein in his arm, and retaining his blood in a large bowl. He consented at once to my proposal. I then requested Dr. Hirtshorn, the resident physician and apothecary of the hospital, to tie up his arm, and bleed him to death. The Doctor instantly feigned a compliance with this request. After losing nearly twenty ounces of blood, he fainted, became calm, and slept soundly the ensuing night. The next day, when I visited him, he was sail unhappy; not from despair and a hatred of life, but from a dread of death; for he now complained only, that several persons in the hospital had conspired to kill him. By the continuance of depleting remedies, this error was removed, and he was soon afterwards discharged from the hospital.

It will naturally occur to the reader, that this remedy, and the use of wine, should be regulated by a strict attention to the state of the pulse.

3. A maniac in the Pennsylvania Hospital, some years ago, expressed a strong desire to drown himself. Mr. Higgins, the present steward of the hos-

pital, seemed to favour this wish, and prepared water for the purpose. The distressed man stripped himself and eagerly jumped into it. Mr. Higgins endeavoured to plunge his head under the water, in order, he said, to hasten his death. The maniac resisted, and declared he would prefer being burnt to death. "You shall be gratified," said Mr. Higgins, and instantly applied a lighted candle to his flesh. "Stop, stop," said he, "I will not die now;" and never afterwards attempted to destroy himself, — or even expressed a wish, for death.

It has been said that persons who make unsuccessful attempts to destroy themselves, seldom repeat them. If this remark be true, I suspect it is only in those cases in which the attempt, like the one above mentioned, has been accompanied with pain.

4. The famous actress Mrs. Bellamy, in an hour of despair, was restrained from suicide by hearing the cry of distress from a child, near a bridge from whence she was preparing to throw herself into the river Thames.

5. Mr. Pinel mentions an instance of a gentleman who was kept from drowning himself in the same river, by an attempt of two or three ruffians to pick his pocket, and which he defeated by a singular exertion of strength and courage.

6. Zacutus relates the history of a hypochondriac who had made several unsuccessful attempts to destroy himself by fire. His physician, in order to cure him, wrapped him in a fresh sheepskin, which he had previously wetted with spirit of turpentine. He applied fire to this skin, which instantly enveloped him in a blaze, that so terrified him, that he never attempted afterwards to put an end to his life.

7. Suicide was prevented in the virgins of Miletus, among whom it was common from the influence of a new and false opinion in religion, by exposing their naked bodies in a public part of the city.

8. Dr. John Hunter tells us, in his account of the diseases of Jamaica, that the negroes, when they become deranged, sometimes destroy themselves by eating large quantities of earth. After many fruitless attempts to put a stop to it, it was finally prevented, by cutting off the heads of the negroes who died in this manner, and exposing them to view in a public part of the Island.

Sometimes patients in this state of derangement destroy themselves by abstinence from food and drinks. I have twice seen death induced in this way in the Pennsylvania Hospital, and once in a private patient. Persuasion and force were alike ineffectual in prevailing upon them to take nourishment. Perhaps some such means as the following might be more effectual for that purpose.

1. In the Memoirs of Count Maurepas, it is related of the same prince of Bourbon who fancied himself to be a plant, that he sometimes supposed himself to be dead, at which time he refused to take any food, for which he said he had no further occasion. To cure this alarming delusion, they contrived to disguise two persons who were introduced to him as his grandfather, and

Marshal Luxemburg, and who, after conversing with him for some time about the shades that inhabited the place of the dead, invited him to dine with marshal Turene. The prince followed them into a cellar prepared for the purpose, where he made a hearty meal, which immediately restored him to a belief that he was alive. A similar case of a man being cured of a belief that he was dead, by being prevailed upon to eat, is related by Dr. Turner, in his Treatise upon the Diseases of the Skin.

2. Mr. Pinel mentions an instance of a man who determined to put an end to his life by abstinence from food only, but who continued to drink as usual. His attendants withheld drinks from him until he consented to take food with them. The bodily pain of thirst, in this case, predominated over the anguish of his mind, which had disposed him to seek for death in this mode of suicide,

3. Leaving food in a patient's cell, or room, and carefully avoiding importuning him to eat. The constant sight of food will tend to excite his appetite, and a consciousness that he possesses his free agency may induce him to eat, when the most powerful arguments for that purpose would not have that effect. I have heard of a criminal in Scotland who attempted to destroy himself by famine, in whom it was completely prevented by this practice.

It is a singular fact in the history of suicide, that it has sometimes been hereditary in families. There are two families in Pennsylvania, in which three of their respective branches have perished by their own hands, in the course of a few years. Similar instances of this issue of family derangement are to be met with in other countries.

In watching patients so as to prevent their injuring, or destroying themselves, it is of importance to know that the paroxysm of despair that prompts to both often comes on suddenly, and is sometimes preceded by unusual tranquility of mind, and even by high spirits.

Chapter Four - Of Amenomania, or the second form of Partial Intellectual Derangement

This form of madness is a higher grade of hypochondriasis, and often succeeds it. It differs from it,

1. In the absence of dyspepsia, or in its cessation, inconsequence of the increase of morbid excitement in the brain, predominating over that disease in the stomach.

2. In a difference, or change, of the patient's opinions respecting his health, affairs and condition. Instead of supposing himself to be diseased, he now denies that he has any disease; and instead of feeling, or complaining of misery, he is now happy in the errors which accompany his madness.

3. The errors in this form of derangement are more deeply seated than in hypochondriasm. As a proof of this, we observe, when it arises from love, the sight, or possession of the object beloved relieves or causes it in the latter

disease, but it has no effect in the former. I have seen it tried to no purpose in a young gentleman in this city. Dr. Nicholas Robinson mentions an instance, in which even the marriage of a young woman to the man whom she loved was so far from curing her, that she attempted to murder him immediately afterwards.

Let it not be supposed that amenomania uniformly succeeds hypochondriasis. It often precedes it, and they both frequently blend their symptoms together. They likewise alternate with each other. There is moreover, now and then, a mixture of some of the symptoms of hysteria with amenomania, as well as with hypochondriasis. These successive changes and combinations of those forms of disease are to be ascribed to irritability or inirritability being different in the systems in which they are seated, and, in some instances, to their being different in different parts of the same system.

Amenomania is a common form of partial insanity. We see it in the enthusiastic votaries of all the pursuits and arts of man. The alchymists, the searchers after perpetual motion, the astronomers, the metaphysicians, the politicians, the knight errants, and the travellers, have all in their turns furnished cases of this form of derangement. I once met with a striking instance of it, from alchymical pursuits, in a gentleman, at the table of Mr. Wolfe, in London. He related the issue of several experiments, in which some of the base metals had been converted into gold, and he declared, further, his belief that there was at that time a man living in India, whose life had been prolonged above 600 years by an elixir that had been discovered by an alchymist. Upon other subjects he was rational and well informed. Dr. Johnson has given a just picture of this disease in the character of an astronomer, in his Rasselas, prince of Abyssinia. Several of the nations of Europe have lately furnished instances of men deranged, from a belief in the possibility of producing perfection in human nature, and in civil government, by means of what they absurdly called the omnipotence of human reason. But we see this disease of the mind most frequently in the enthusiasts in religion, in whom it discovers itself in a variety of ways; particularly,

1. In a belief that they are the peculiar favourites of heaven, and exclusively possessed of just opinions of the divine will, as revealed in the Scriptures.

2. That they see and converse with angels, and the departed spirits of their relations and friends.

3. That they are favoured with visions, and the revelation of future events. And,

4. That they are exalted into beings of the highest order. I have seen two instances of persons, who believed themselves to be the Messiah, and I have heard of each of the sacred names and offices of the Father, Son, and Holy Ghost, having been assumed at the same time by three persons, under the influence of this partial form of derangement, in a hospital in Mexico.

There was a time when persons thus deranged were subjected to fines, imprisonment, the extirpation of their tongues, and even to death from fire and the halter. To the influence of the science of medicine we are indebted, for teaching that these opinions are generally as devoid of impiety as an epileptic fit; and for consigning, by that humane discovery, the deluded subjects of them to the cells of a hospital instead of a jail, and to the hand of a physician, instead of the hands of the last officer, of what has improperly been called, criminal justice.

In all these cases of partial derangement, the understanding is not only sound upon subjects unconnected with that which produced the disease, but all the other faculties of the mind are unimpaired; nor do we observe the subjects of it, as in general madness, to be irritated, or unusually excited, by conversing upon the single and original subject of their disease.

It is remarkable that all the errors of amenomania are the reverse of those of tristimania, formerly mentioned, in elevating the patient above his ordinary rank and condition of life.

The physical remedies for this form of partial derangement are nearly the same as those which have been recommended for tristimania, particularly bleeding, purging, emetics, and low diet, in an excited state of the blood-vessels, and, after they are reduced, stimulating diet, drinks and medicines, and a change of company, pursuits, and climate. The errors which predominate in the mind should be soothed, diverted, or opposed by reasoning or ridicule, according to their force. There is one error which is sometimes opposed by reasoning with success, and that is, a belief, which patients in this pleasant state of derangement now and then entertain, that they are favoured with extraordinary revelations, and particularly a knowledge of future events. In these cases they should be told, that supernatural knowledge of that kind; has generally been revealed to two or more persons at the same time, and that it has always been accompanied with a power of working miracles. Even the Saviour of the world did not rest the credibility of his divine origin, and the objects of his mission, upon his single testimony in favour of himself, nor yet upon the supreme and miraculous power he exercised over spirit and matter; but condescended to receive the testimony of his twelve apostles in favour of the former, and compelled a belief in the latter, by endowing them with a power, similar to his own, over all the operations of nature.

Both tristimania and amenomania often continue for months and years, in the form in which they have been described, but they are as often followed by derangement in every part of the understanding, and in all, or a part of, the other faculties of the mind. When this is the case, it is called general madness, which is the next subject of our inquiries and observations.

Chapter Five - Of General Intellectual Derangement

I shall divide this general form of derangement into three grades or states.

I. **Mania,** by which I mean what has been called tonic madness by some writers, and mania furibunda by Vanswieten.

II. **Manicula,** or madness in a reduced, and most commonly in a chronic, state.

III. **Manalgia,** or that state of general madness, in which a universal torpor takes place in the body and mind.

This division of general madness into three states, accords with similar divisions, which have lately been adopted of several other diseases, particularly rheumatism, and inflammation of the liver. The former is known by the names of rheumatismus, rheumaticula, and rheumatalgia, and the latter by the names of hepatitis, hepaticula, and hepitalgia. The propriety of thus conforming madness to the divisions of those two diseases will appear when we consider the unity of their proximate cause, and that they all depend upon similar morbid actions in the blood-vessels. Rheumatism and hepatitis, therefore, may be considered, if I may be allowed the illustration, as madness in the joints, or liver; and madness, as rheumatism, or hepatitis, in the brain.

I. I shall begin with the history and cure of general madness of the first grade, or of what I have called **mania**. Its premonitory signs are, watchfulness, high or low spirits, great rapidity of thought, and eccentricity in conversation, and conduct; sometimes pathetic expressions of horror, excited by the apprehension of approaching madness; terrifying or distressing dreams; great irritability of temper; jealousy; instability in all pursuits; unusual acts of extravagance, manifested by the purchases of houses, and certain expensive and unnecessary articles of furniture, and hostility to relations and friends. The face is pale or flushed, the eyes are dull, or wild, the appetite is increased, the bowels are costive, and the patient complains sometimes of throbbing in the temples, vertigo, and head-ache. The gentleman formerly mentioned, in whom madness was excited by a number of small shot lodged in his foot, when a school boy was afflicted with deafness. A sudden return of his hearing was always a premonitory sign of an approaching attack of derangement.

The remedies in this case should be,

1. The removal of all the remote and exciting causes of the disease, and particularly to abstract the patient from study and business, if they have produced it, and to substitute in their room relaxation and amusements. Dr. Boerhaave once passed several weeks without sleep, and discovered other signs of approaching derangement. He was cured by being torn from his books, and allured into agreeable company.

2. Changing the subjects of our patients studies, when they are abstruse and difficult, to such as are of a lighter nature. Rousseau often removed, by this means, the premonitory symptoms of madness. The celebrated Mr.

M'Laurin, the friend and cotemporary of sir Isaac Newton, made it a practice to relieve his mind, when debilitated by hard study, and thereby predisposed to this disease, by reading novels and romances; and such was his knowledge of them, that the late Dr. Gregory informed me he was often appealed to for the character of every work of that kind that appeared in the English language.

3. Low diet, and a few gentle doses of purging physic, and, if the pulse be full or tense, the loss of ten or twelve ounces of blood. By means of these remedies, I have in many instances prevented an attack of madness.

The symptoms of this state of derangement, when completely formed, as they appear in the body, are, a wild and ferocious countenance, enlarged and rolling eyes, constant singing, whistling or hallowing, imitation of the noises of different animals, walking with a quick step, or standing still, often with the hands and eyes elevated towards the heavens; wakefulness for whole nights, weeks, months, and, according to Dr. Morely's account of a boy at Naples, for years; great muscular strength, uncommon adroitness in performing certain acts, and uncommon swiftness in running. The nerves are insensible to cold, heat, and to irritants of all kinds. I am aware that insensibility to cold is denied by Mr. Halsam to be a symptom of general madness. I admit that it does not take place in one of its states, that is, in manicula, but it is uniformly present, as I shall prove by facts hereafter, in its highest and lowest grades, in which states the system resists not only cold and heat, but all the usual remote causes of fever from the insensible qualities of the atmosphere. Sometimes the nerves exhibit, in great mobility, several of the signs of hysteria mixed with general madness. The chief of these signs are laughing and weeping. They occur oftener in women than men.

The skin is dry, cool, and sometimes covered with profuse sweats. A coldness often affects the feet only, for days and weeks, while the head, and other parts of the body, are preternaturally warm, or of their natural temperature

The senses of hearing and seeing are uncommonly acute. This is obvious, from their hearing so distinctly low and distant sounds, and from their prompt recollection of long unseen and forgotten faces, and of the resemblance of persons, whom they have never seen before, to their parents, or to some other of their ancestors'.

The tongue is generally moist, and frequently has a whitish appearance, such as occurs in common fevers. There is sometimes a preternatural secretion of saliva and mucus in the mouth and throat, which is of a viscid nature, and discharged with difficulty by spitting. From the constancy of this symptom in some mad people, they obtained the name of sputatores, or spitters. There is generally a stoppage of the secretion of mucus in the nose. - Dr. Moore found this to be the case in two thirds of all the maniacs in the Pennsylvania Hospital, whom he examined at my request, with a reference to this symptom. Where this secretion was not suspended, he found the mucus of the nose dry and hard.

The appetite for food is great, or there is a total want of it. The bowels are generally costive, and the stools white, small, and hard. The urine is scanty in quantity, and, for the most part, of a high colour.

The pulse is synocha, intermitting, preternaturally slow, frequent, quick, depressed, or morbidly natural, exactly as we find it in other arterial diseases of great morbid action. It is generally depressed, where the muscles are in a state of violent excitement.

The symptoms of mania, as they appear in the mind, vary with its causes. When it is induced by impressions that have been made upon the brain through the medium of the heart, all the faculties of the mind discover marks of the disease in all their operations. In its highest grade, it produces erroneous perception. In this state of derangement, the patient mistakes the persons and objects around him , This may arise either from a disease in the external senses, in which case it is called morbid sensation; or from a disease in the brain. It is when it arises from the latter cause only, a symptom of the first or highest grade of intellectual derangement. We have a striking illustration of this diseased state of perception in the character of Ajax, in the tragedy of Sophocles. He becomes mad, in consequence of Ulysses being preferred to him in the competition for the arms of Achilles. In one of his paroxysms of madness, he runs into the fields, and slays a number of shepherds and their cattle, under a belief that they were Agamemnon, Menelaus, and others, who had been the instruments of his dishonour. Afterwards he brings a number of cattle to his tent, and among them a large ram, which he puts to death for his rival and antagonist Ulysses. Persons under the influence of this grade of madness sometimes mistake their friends for strangers, and common visitors for their relations and friends. They now and then fancy they see good or bad spirits standing by their bed-sides, waiting to carry them to a place of torment or happiness, according as their moral dispositions and habits in health have prepared them for those different abodes of wicked or pious souls. Not only the eyes, but the ears likewise, are the vehicles of false perceptions, and to these we are to ascribe the soliloquies we sometimes observe in mad people. They fancy they are spoken to, and their conversation frequently consists of replies only to certain questions they suppose to be put to them. These false perceptions are more common through the ears than the eyes in mad people. The latter occur constantly more or less in delirium, but we occasionally see them in the highest grade of intellectual madness. When these errors in perception take place, madness has been called *ideal* by Dr. Arnold, but more happily, *diseased* perception by Dr. Creighton. It is in this state of madness only that it is proper to say, persons are "out of their senses;" for the mind no longer receives the true images of external objects from them.

To account for these erroneous or diseased perceptions, it will be necessary to remark, that the correspondence of ideas and thoughts with impressions, depends upon the *sameness* of the impressions which produced the original ideas and thoughts. Now this correspondence can take place only when the brain is in a healthy state. When it is *diseased,* impressions induce unrelated ideas and thoughts, as in the case of Ajax just now mentioned. It will be necessary to remark further in this place, that no idea can be excited in the mind, however erroneous it may be, from a want of relation between impression and perception, that did not pre-exist in the mind. Ajax could not have fancied a large ram to be Ulysses, had not his image from a former impression of his person upon his brain, pre-existed in his mind; and it was because the part of his brain which was stimulated by the image of the ram did not emit a corresponding perception, but conveyed the motion excited by it to that part of the brain in which the image of Ulysses had been imprinted, that he saw him instead of a ram. The nature of this error of perception may be understood, by recollecting how often impressions upon a sound part of the body produce sensation and motion, in parts that are affected with a morbid sensibility and irritability, that are remote from it. These errors, as applied to the body, have lately received the names of error sensus, and error motus. They occur in all the senses, as well as in the nerves, muscles and brain.

Where these erroneous perceptions do not take place, the associations of a madman are often discordant, ludicrous, or offensive, and his judgment and reason are perverted upon all subjects. He sometimes attempts to injure himself or others. Even inanimate objects, such as his clothing, bed, chairs, tables, and the windows, doors, and walls of his room, when confined, partake of his rage. All sense of decency and modesty is suspended; hence he besmears his face with his own excretions, and exposes his whole body without a covering. When he roams at large, or escapes from a place of confinement, lonely woods, marshes, caves, or grave-yards, are his usual places of resort, or retirement. What is called consciousness is at this time destroyed in his mind. He is ignorant of the place he occupies, and of his rank and condition in society, of the lapse of time, and even of his own personal identity. Shakespeare has very happily described a part of this state of mind, when he makes King Lear utter the following words:

> --------------------"I am mainly ignorant
> What place this is; and all the skill I have
> Remembers not these garments, nor I know not
> Where I did sleep last night."

This grade of derangement is generally of short duration. It gradually leaves the memory, and appears with less force in the passions and moral faculties, but still occupies, in a greater or less degree, every part of the understanding.

The sameness in the operations of nature, in thus gradually contracting the seat and extent of this disease to one faculty of the mind, and in contracting the seat and extent of violent fevers to the blood-vessels, was noticed in a former part of these Inquiries.

In this reduced state of madness, the mind becomes more coherent, and perceives, and associates correctly, but judges incorrectly, that is, draws erroneous conclusions from false premises. But there are cases in this reduced grade of derangement in which the patient perceives justly, associates naturally, judges correctly, but reasons erroneously, that is, draws false conclusions from just prepositions. Sometimes he discovers the reverse of this state of mind, by drawing just conclusions from erroneous perceptions, associations and judgments. Thus, when he fancies himself to be a king, he errs in all the ways that have been mentioned. But observe his conduct: he covers himself with a blanket which he calls a robe, he puts a mat upon his head which he calls a crown, struts with a majestic step, and demands the homage due to royalty from all around him. In this respect he reasons justly from false premises, and acts conformably to the high opinion he entertains of his rank and power. In a more advanced state of the disease, the hostility of the patient is confined to his friends and relations only, and this is frequently great in proportion to the nearness of the connection, and the extent of the obligations he owes to them. Its intensity cannot be conceived of by persons who have observed that passion only in ordinary life. I once advised a ride in a chair, for one of my private patients in this state of mind, in the Pennsylvania Hospital. Before he got into it, he made the steward of the hospital, who was to accompany him, declare, that no one of his family had ever rode in it. But further, while the disease occupies the whole understanding, the patient discovers more derangement in talking upon some subjects than others. These subjects are sometimes of a pleasant, but oftener of a distressing nature. The disease varies with each of them by putting on the appearance of amenomania in the former, and tristimania in the latter case. It differs from them both in the errors and prejudices that are entertained by the patient, being accompanied with more corporeal and mental excitement; in being less fixed to one object, and in occupying every part of the understanding.

From a part of the brain being preternaturally elevated, but not diseased, the mind sometimes discovers not only unusual strength and acuteness, but certain talents it never exhibited before. The records of the wit and cunning of madmen are numerous in every country. Talents for eloquence, poetry, music and painting, and uncommon ingenuity in several of the mechanical arts, are often evolved in this state of madness. A gentleman whom I attended in our hospital in the year 1810 often delighted, as well as astonished, the patients and officers of our hospital, by his displays of oratory, in preaching from a table in the hospital yard every Sunday. A female patient of mine, who became insane after parturition in the year 1807, sang hymns and songs, of her own composition, during the latter stage of her illness, with a tone of voice so soft and pleasant, that I hung upon it with delight, every time I visited her. She had never discovered a talent for poetry nor music in any previous part of her life. Two instances of a talent for drawing, evolved by madness, have occurred within my knowledge; and where is the hospital for mad people, in which elegant and completely rigged ships, and curious pieces of machinery, have not been exhibited, by persons who never discovered the least turn for a mechanical art previously to their derangement. Sometimes we observe in mad people an unexpected resuscitation of knowledge; hence we hear them describe past events, and speak in ancient or modern languages, or repeat long and interesting passages from books, none of which we are sure they were capable of recollecting, in the natural and healthy state of their minds.

The disease which thus evolves these new and wonderful talents and operations of the mind may be compared to an earthquake, which, by convulsing the upper strata of our globe, throws upon its surface precious and splendid fossils, the existence of which was unknown to the proprietors of the soil in which they were buried.

Sometimes the cause which induced derangement is forgotten, and the subjects of the ravings, as well as the conduct of patients, are contrary to their usual habits; but they both more frequently accord with their natural tempers and dispositions, and with the cause of their disease.

Are they naturally proud and ambitious? They imagine themselves to be kings, or noblemen, and demand homage and respect. Are they naturally avaricious? They fancy they possess incalculable wealth. Are they ferocious and malicious? They assume the nature of wild beasts, and attempt to injure their friends and keepers. Are they sensual and slovenly in their dispositions and dress? They discover marks of both in their conversation and appearance? Are they pious and benevolent? They are inoffensive in their deportment, and spend much time in devotional exercises. - But the conduct and language of madmen are much influenced by the specific cause that induces it. Does it arise from reciprocal love, opposed in the object of mutual wishes by interested friends? It vents itself in sighs and songs, or sonnets and love letters. Is madness induced by perfidy in a lover? It discovers itself in all the usual marks of resentment, rage, and, when practicable, of revenge. Ariosto has with great elegance and correctness described these marks in the conduct of Orlando, when deserted by his beloved Angelica. He lies down upon a bed in order to rest a few minutes, but the moment he recollects that Angelica once slept upon that bed, he instantly starts from it, tears up the tree by the roots upon which she had cut her name, and finally dries up the water in which she had been accustomed to view her face.

Has the disease been induced by a conflict between the moral faculty, and the sexual appetite, or by the undue gratification of it? The habitual and morbid impurity of the mind discovers itself in corresponding conversations and actions. Several cases of this kind in both sexes, have occurred in our hospital.

But, further, is madness induced by the ingratitude or treachery of friends, or by the unjust calumnies of the world? the conversation and conduct of the patient indicate a coldness or hostility to the whole human race. In this state of mind, the walls of a cell, and even darkness, are welcomed, to protect the miserable sufferer from the sight of the supposed monster — man.

Mr. Merry has very forcibly described the feelings of a person deranged from this cause, in the following lines:

"By sharp sensation wounded to the soul,
He ponders on the world; abhors the whole.
In the dire working of his wakeful dreams,
The human race a race of demons seems.
All is unjust, discordant and severe;
He asks not mercy's smile, nor pity's tear.

Is it induced by misfortunes in business, and by the rapacity and cruelty of creditors? He sees a sheriff, or one of his deputies, in every person that opens his door, and talks of nothing but of the horrors of a jail. Mr. Merry has described this state of mind likewise, with great correctness, in the following lines.

"But most to him shall memory prove a curse,
Who meets capricious fortune's sad reverse.
Who once, in wealth, indulg'd each gay desire,
While to possess, was only to require.
Who scatter'd bounty with a liberal hand,
And rov'd, at will, through pleasure's flow'ry land.
By ruin cast amongst the lowly crew,
What doleful visions pass before his view!
His taste, his worth, his wisdom disappear,
His virtues, too, none notice, none revere.
Cold is the summer friend, who liv'd to trace
His playful fancy's ever varying grace.
Even nature's self a different aspect wears,
Dimm'd by the mists of slow consuming cares.
Glows not a flower, nor pants a vernal breeze.
As in his hours of affluence and ease.
While every luxury that the world displays
Wounds him afresh, and tells of better days."

Is madness induced by remorse for real or imaginary crimes? The wretched sufferer fancies his bedroom a dungeon, and his physician an executioner, or he cries out to be delivered from infernal spirits, which he supposes to be waiting around his bed, to carry his soul to a place of torment.

Is it induced by false and gloomy opinions of the attributes of the Deity, and a belief of being destined to endless misery? His apartment becomes vocal day and night with the groans and sighs, and the excruciating language of despair.

Is it brought on by a belief in his being a peculiar favourite of heaven, and destined to fulfil some of its high and benevolent decrees? His mind overflows with enthusiastic joy, and he stands aloof from an intercourse, and even from the contact of mortals. Two instances of this kind have come under my knowledge in this city.

Has the sudden and unexpected acquisition of great wealth perverted the natural operations of the mind? The maniac from this cause is elevated, cheerful, sings and laughs from morning till night. I have seen one instance of this state of madness in our hospital from the cause I have mentioned. It is from such cases of madness, that it has been said to be attended with pleasure. Horace's madman complained of his physician, for restoring him to his former humble grade of life by curing him, and Dr. Thomas Willis mentions an instance of a man, who was so happy in his paroxysms of madness, that when he was well he longed with impatience for their return; but such instances of happiness in madness are very rare. It is more frequently, I shall say hereafter, accompanied with misery, or a total insensibility to it.

The nature of a paroxysm of madness is much diversified, by its affecting the moral faculties, or leaving them in a sound state. Shakespeare has happily illustrated the encroachment of intellectual madness upon the moral faculty, and the sudden recovery of its correct state, in the following lines, which he makes his mad King Lear to utter upon being called upon to punish one of his subjects for adultery.

"Thou shalt not die — die for adultery!
No! — to it luxury — pell mell —
For I want soldiers."

And then, as if suddenly penetrated with a sense of the indecency of what he had said, he adds,

"Fie! — Fie! — Fie! — Pah!
Give me an ounce of civet, good apothecary,
To sweeten my imagination."

The reader will excuse my frequent references to the poets for facts to illustrate the history of madness. They view the human mind in all its operations, whether natural or morbid, with a microscopic eye; and hence many things arrest their attention, which escape the notice of physicians.

To the history that has been given of the correspondence between the ravings and conduct of mad people, and their natural tempers and dispositions, there are several exceptions. These are, all those cases in which persons of exemplary piety and purity of character utter profane, or impious, or indelicate language, and behave in other respects contrary to their moral habits. The apparent vices of such deranged people may be compared to the offensive substances that are sometimes thrown upon the surface of the globe by an earthquake, mixed with the splendid fossils formerly mentioned, which substances had no existence in nature, but were formed by a new arrange-

64

ment in the particles of matter in consequence of the violent commotions in the bowels of the earth.

Not only the ravings of mad people, for the most part, accord with their habitual tempers and dispositions, and the causes of their disease, but their conduct corresponds in like manner with their habitual occupations. The lawyer, the physician, and the minister of the gospel, frequently employ themselves in the exercises of their several professions. The merchant spends much of his time in making out invoices, and in writing letters; the politician devours a daily news-paper; the poet writes verses; and the painter draws pictures upon the walls of their respective cells; the mechanic cuts out houses, ships, carriages, and bridges, from pieces of sticks, with his pen-knife; the sailor heaves his log or his line; and the soldier goes through his manual exercise with a cane, and never fails to salute his visitors by lifting the back of his hand to the side of his head.

These habitual actions seldom take place until the disease has subsided, in a considerable degree, in the temper and passions.

After the detail of the symptoms of general madness that has been given, I feel disposed to look back for a few minutes, and contemplate, with painful and melancholy wonder, the immense changes in the human mind, that are induced by a little alteration in the circulation of the blood in the brain. What great effects are produced in this instance by little causes! How slender the tenure by which we hold our intellectual and moral existence! and how humiliating our situation from its loss! Well might the eloquent Mr. Cowper, from this view of the mind of man, consider it as

------- "A harp, whose chords elude the sight,
Each yielding harmony, dispos'd aright.
The screws revers'd! (A task, which, if he please,
God in a moment executes with ease)
Ten thousand times ten thousand strings go loose:
Lost! till he tune them, all their power and use."

There is a considerable variety in the forms of general madness. It appears,

I. In a *single,* acute and violent paroxysm, such as has been described, which continues for days, weeks, and sometimes months, and ends in death, a remission, or a perfect and durable recovery. In one of the cases of a protracted paroxysm of madness which came under my notice, the disease continued from June 1810 until April 1811, with scarcely any abatement in the excitement of the body and mind, notwithstanding the patient was constantly under the operation of depleting remedies. I have seen another case, in which the same remedies were insufficient to produce an interruption of five minutes of speech or vociferations, except during a few short intervals of sleep, for two months.

II. General madness appears in a chronic but more moderate form, without paroxyms.

65

III. It appears with paroxysms, with chronic, but moderate, derangement in its intervals. In these intervals, the patient sometimes recovers so far as so discover derangement upon one subject only. In these cases, a return of general madness is easily excited at any time, by touching upon the subject of his partial insanity in conversing with him. Thus the touch of one of the cords of a musical instrument causes all its cords to vibrate with it. In this, I remarked formerly, general madness differs from the two forms of partial madness which have been described.

IV. It appears in paroxysms, with the restoration of reason in their intervals. These paroxysms occur annually, or at longer intervals, twice a year, particularly during the equinoxes, monthly, weekly, and according to Lazoni, an Italian physician, every day. Perhaps this diurnal attack of madness was what has lately been called the maniacal state of fever.

Successive paroxysms of madness, with perfect intervals between them, occur most frequently in habitual drunkards; and they would probably occur much oftener, were they not prevented by a vicarious affection of the stomach, known by puking, redness of the eyes, an active pulse, and a peculiar and specific foetor of the breath. From the correspondence of several of the actions which take place in this disease of the stomach, with those which take place in the brain in madness, and from the sameness of the ordinary duration of a paroxysm of each of them, I have called the former, derangement in the stomach.

The longer the intervals between the paroxysms of madness, the more complete is the restoration of reason. Remissions, rather than intermissions, take place when the intervals are of short duration, and these distinguish it from febrile delirium, in which intermissions more generally occur. In many cases, every thing is remembered that passes under the notice of the patient during a paroxysm of general madness, but in those cases in which the memory is diseased, as well as the understanding, nothing is recollected. I attended a lady, in the month of October 1802, who had crossed the Atlantic Ocean during a paroxysm of derangement, without recollecting a single circumstance of her voyage, any more than if she had passed the whole time in sleep. Sometimes every thing is forgotten in the interval of a paroxysm, but recollected in a succeeding paroxysm, I once attended the daughter of a British officer, who had been educated in the habits of gay life, who was married to a Methodist minister. In her paroxysms of madness she resumed her gay habits, spoke French, and ridiculed the tenets and practices of the sect to which she belonged. In the intervals of her fits she renounced her gay habits, became zealously devoted to the religious principles and ceremonies of the Methodists, and forgot everything she did and said during the fits of her insanity. A deranged sailor, some years ago in the Pennsylvania Hospital, fancied himself to be an admiral, and walked and commanded with all the dignity and authority that are connected with that high rank in the navy. He was cured and discharged: his disease some time after wards returned, and with it all the actions of an admiral which he assumed and imitated in his former paroxysm. It is remarkable, some persons when deranged talk *rationally,* but act *irrationally,* while others act *rationally* and talk *irrationally.* We had a sailor some years ago in our hospital, who spent a whole year in building and rigging a small ship in his cell. Every part of it was formed by a mind apparently in a sound state. During the whole of the year in which he was employed in this work, he spoke not a word. In bringing his ship out of his cell, a part of it was broken. He immediately spoke, and became violently deranged soon afterwards. Again, some madmen *talk* rationally, and *write* irrationally; but it is more common for them to utter a few connected sentences in conversation, but not to be able to connect two correct sentences together in a letter. Of this I have known many instances in our hospital.

V. Mania is sometimes combined with phrenitis. The brain in this case is in the same state, as the lungs when an acute pneumony blends itself with a pulmonary consumption. Excitement in both cases is abstracted from the muscles, so that the patients are usually confined to their beds. The tongue is more furred, and the skin much warmer, in this mixture of mania and phrenitis, than in madness alone. It occurs most frequently after parturition. I have taken the liberty of calling it *Phrenimania.*

VI. Mania is sometimes combined with the burning-, sweating, cold, chilly, intermitting, and even hydrophobic states of fever. Instances of them were mentioned in treating upon the seat and proximate cause of madness. A case of its union with hydrophobia occurred in a lady under my care in the month of February 1812. She attempted several times to bite her attendants, and was greatly agitated when the word "water" was mentioned in her room. As the pulse in this mixture of mania and common fever is generally synochus, I have called it *Synocomania.*

In all the forms and combinations of madness that have been described, the duration of the disease, after it is completely formed, seems to be as much fixed by nature as the duration of an autumnal fever. It may be weakened, and life may be preserved during its continuance, but, unless it be overcome in its first stage, it generally runs its course, in spite of all the power of medicine.

VII. There is a form of mania which is seldom the object of medical attention, either in hospitals, or in private practice, but which is well known, not only to physicians, but to persons of common observation in every part of the world. Dr. Cox has described it very happily and correctly in the following words.

"Among the varieties of maniacs met with in medical practice, there is one, which, though by no means rare, has been little noticed by writers on this subject: I refer to those cases, in which the individuals perform most of the common duties of life with propriety, and some of them, indeed, with scrupulous exactness; who exhibit no strongly marked features of either temperament, no traits of superior or defective mental endowment, but yet take violent antipathies, harbour unjust suspicions, indulge strong propensities, affect singularity in dress, gait, and phraseology; are proud, conceited, and ostentatious; easily excited, and with difficulty appeased; dead to sensibility, delicacy, and refinement; obstinately riveted to the most absurd opinions; prone to controversy, and yet incapable of reasoning; always the hero of their own tale, using hyperbolic high-flown language to express the most simple ideas, accompanied by unnatural gesticulation, inordinate action, and frequently by the most alarming expression of countenance. On some occasions they suspect similar intentions on the most trivial grounds, on others are a prey to fear and dread from the most ridiculous and imaginary sources; now embracing every opportunity of exhibiting romantic courage and feats of hardihood, then indulging themselves in all manner of excesses.

"Persons of this description, to the casual observer, might appear actuated by a bad heart, but the experienced physician knows it is the head which is defective. They seem as if constantly affected by a greater or less degree Of stimulation from intoxicating liquors, while the expression of countenance furnishes an infallible proof of mental disease. If subjected to moral restraint, or a medical regimen, they yield with reluctance to the means proposed, and generally refuse and resist, on the ground that such means are unnecessary where no disease exists; and when, by the system adopted, they are so far recovered, as to be enabled to suppress the exhibition of the former peculiarities, and are again fit to be restored to society, the physician, and those friends who put them under the physician's care, are generally ever after objects of enmity, and frequently of revenge."

VIII. There is a form of madness which is altogether *internal,* and of which I have met with several instances. It consists in the same kind of alienation of mind that takes place in common madness, but which is subject to the command of the will: persons affected with it feel all the distraction of thoughts and anguish of madness when alone, and sometimes in company, when they are silent, or inattentive to conversation, but without discovering any of its signs in their countenances or behaviour. It resembles, in this respect, that feeble grade of the delirium of a fever, which is chased away by the visit of a physician, or by speaking to the patient upon any interesting subject. I have suspected the cases of suicide, which sometimes occur in persons apparently in a sound state of mind, are occasioned by this form of madness. They may be compared, in this situation, to patients in the walking state of the yellow fever, in whom all the sympathies of the body are destroyed, in consequence of which its external parts appear sound and healthy, while the stomach, and other vital parts are perishing by disease. I have called this internal form of madness *mania larvata.*

There has been a diversity of opinions respecting the influence of the moon in inducing, or increasing, paroxysms of madness, after it has taken possession of the system. The late Dr. James Hutchinson, who spent several years in the Pennsylvania hospital as its resident physician and apothecary, assured me, that he had never seen the least change in the disease of the maniacs from the state of the moon. Mr. Halsam tells us, that in two years close attention to the state of the maniacs in Bethlehem Hospital, in London, he had never seen their disease increase at the lunar periods. To these facts is opposed the testimony of ages, in all countries. There is, I believe, an equal portion of truth on the side of both these opinions. In order to reconcile them, it will be proper to remark, 1st, that in certain diseases and in certain debilitated states of the system, the body acquires a kind of *sixth* sense, that is, a perception of heat and cold, of moisture and dryness, of the density and rarity of the air, and of light and darkness, of which it is insensible in a healthy state. 2, The moon, when full, increases the rarity of the air and the quantity of light, each of which I believe acts upon sick people in various diseases, and, among others, in madness. A predisposition to the action of such feeble causes is required in all cases. From the conversion of excitability into excitement in mania, and from its absence in manalgia, it is easy to conceive, in both those states of derangement, the system will be insensible to the influence of the moon. Now when we consider that a great majority of the patients in most hospitals are in one of those states of madness, it is easy to account for their exhibiting no marks of lunar influence, according to the observations of Dr. Hutchinson and Mr. Halsam. In the year 1807 I requested Mr. Thornton, then one of the apothecaries of the hospital, to attend particularly to the influence of the morning light upon all the maniacal patients that were at that time confined in it. He informed me, that many of them became noisy as soon as the day began to break, and that, with the exception of two or three recent cases, they all became silent and quiet after night. During the eclipse of the sun on the 16th of June 1806, there was a sudden and total silence in all the cells of the hospital.

The inference from these facts is, that the cases are few in which mad people feel the influence of the moon, and that when they do, it is derived chiefly from an increase of its light. It is possible the absence of its light may be attended with equal commotions in the system of patients who are afflicted with that form of derangement which I have called tristimania.

It is possible, further, that in the few cases in which the light of the moon, or the rarity of the air, is felt by deranged persons in a hospital, that their noise, by keeping a number of patients in neighbouring cells awake, and in a state of inquietude from the want of sleep, may have contributed to establish that general belief in the influence of the moon upon madness, which has so long obtained among physicians.

Chapter Six - Of the Remedies for Mania

Before we proceed to mention the remedies for mania, or the highest grade of general madness, it will be necessary to mention the means of establishing a complete government over patients afflicted with it, and thus, by securing their obedience, respect, and affections, to enable a physician to apply his remedies with ease, certainty and success.

The first thing to be done, to accomplish these purposes, is to remove the patient from his family, and from the society of persons whom he has been accustomed to command, to a place where he will be prevented from injuring himself and others. If there be objections to removing him to a public or private madhouse, or if this be impracticable, the patient should be confined in a chamber, in which he has not been accustomed to sleep, and a stranger or strangers should be employed, exclusively, to attend him. The effect of thus depriving a madman of his liberty has sometimes been of the most salutary nature, by suddenly creating a new current of ideas, as well as by the depression it produces in his mind.

1. This preliminary measure being taken, the first object of a physician, when he enters the cell, or chamber, of his deranged patient, should be, to catch his eye, and look him out of countenance. The dread of the eye was early imposed upon every beast of the field. The tyger, the mad bull, and the enraged dog, all fly from it: now a man deprived of his reason partakes so much of the nature of those animals, that he is for the most part easily terrified, or composed, by the eye of a man who possesses his reason. I know this dominion of the eye over mad people is denied by Mr. Halsam, from his supposing that it consists simply in imparting to the eye a stern or ferocious look. This may sometimes be necessary; but a much greater effect is produced, by looking the patient out of countenance with a mild and steady eye, and varying its aspect from the highest degree of sternness, down to the mildest degree of benignity; for there are keys in the eye, if I may be allowed the expression, which should be suited to the state of the patient's mind, with the same exactness that musical tones should be suited to the depression of spirits in hypochondriasis. - Mr. Halsam again asks, "Where is the man that would trust himself alone with a madman, with no other means of subduing him than by his eye?" This may be, and yet the efficacy of the eye as a calming remedy not be called in question. It is but one of several other remedies that are proper to tranquilize him; and, when used alone, may not be sufficient for th.it purpose. Who will deny the efficacy of bleeding for the cure of madness? and yet who would rely upon it exclusively, without the aid of other remedies? In favour of the power of the eye, in conjunction with other means, in composing mad people, I can speak from the experience of many years. It has been witnessed by several hundred students of medicine in our hospital, and once by several of the managers of the hospital, in the case of a man recently brought into their room, and whose conduct for a considerable time resisted its efficacy.

2. A second means of securing the obedience of a deranged patient to a physician should be by his voice. Milton calls the human face "divine." It would be more proper to apply that epithet to the human voice, from its wonderful effects upon the mind of man, whether employed in simple tones,

in music, or in speech. Even brutes feel and obey it. In governing mad people it should be harsh, gentle, or plaintive, according to circumstances. I have observed with great pleasure the most beneficial effects produced by it in all those ways. A patient in the Pennsylvania Hospital, who called his physician his father, once lifted his hand to strike him. "What!" said his physician, with a plaintive tone of voice, "strike your father!" The madman dropped his arm, and instantly showed marks of contrition for his conduct.

In Java, madness of a furious kind is often brought on by the intemperate use of opium. The poor, when affected with it, are put to death; but the rich, who are able to purchase the services of female nurses, generally recover. May not their recovery be ascribed, in part, to their ears being constantly exposed to the gentleness and softness of a female voice?

3. The countenance of a physician should assist his eye and voice in governing his deranged patients. It should be accommodated to the state of the patient's mind and conduct. There is something like contagion in the different aspects of the human face, and madmen feel it in common with other people. A grave countenance in a physician has often checked the frothy levity of a deranged patient in an instant, and a placid one has as suddenly chased away his gloom. A stern countenance in like manner has often put a stop to garrulity, and a cheerful one has extorted smiles even from the face of melancholy itself.

4. The conduct of a physician to his patients should be uniformly dignified, if he wishes to acquire their obedience and respect. He should never descend to levity in conversing with them. He should hear with silence their rude or witty answers to his questions, and upon no account ever laugh at them, or with them.

5. Acts of justice, and a strict regard to truth, tend to secure the respect and obedience of deranged patients to their physician. Every thing necessary for their comfort should be provided for them, and every promise made to them should be faithfully and punctually performed. I once lost the confidence of a maniac, by simply failing to enlarge him on an appointed day, in consequence of an unexpected revival of some of the symptoms of his disease.

6. A physician should treat his deranged patients with respect, and with all the ceremonies which are due to their former rank and habits of living. Carpets upon the floors of their rooms or cells, curtains to their beds, taste in the preparation and manner of serving their meals, will all serve to prevent distress and irritation, from a supposed change in their condition in life. I have known a deranged gentleman complain of being addressed without the title of Mr.; and I have seen several others turn with an indignant look from their food, when served to them upon a table not covered with a cloth, or in vessels they had not been accustomed to in their own families. With this habitual attachment to forms in behaviour, and taste in living, there is in this class of patients a similar respect for former habits of society, for which reason they should always eat, sit, and partake of amusements, by themselves. The

great advantage which private madhouses have over public hospitals is derived chiefly from their conforming to this principle in human nature; which the highest grade of madness is seldom able to eradicate.

7. And lastly. A physician acquires the obedience and affections of his deranged patients by **acts of kindness**. For this purpose, all his directions for discontinuing painful or disagreeable remedies, and all his pleasant prescriptions, should be delivered in the presence of his patients; while such as are of an unpleasant nature, should be delivered only to their keepers. Small presents of fruit or sweet-cake will have a happy effect in attaching maniacal patients to their physicians, for it is a fact, that in proportion to the intensity of misery, the subjects of it feel most sensibly the smallest diminution of it. Perhaps the recovery of the madmen in Java, just now mentioned, may be ascribed, further, to their being nursed by women, in whom kindness to the sick and distressed is so universal, that it forms an essential and predominating feature in the female character.

As an inducement to treat mad people in the manner that has been recommended, I shall only add, that in those cases in which the memory has been greatly impaired, they seldom forget three things after their recovery, viz. acts of cruelty, acts of indignity, and acts of kindness. I have known instances in which the two former have been recollected by them with painful, and the last with pleasant associations for many years. In gratitude tor kindness and favours shown to them, they exceed all other classes of patients after their recovery. A physician once asked a young woman of the society of Friends, whom he had assisted in curing in the Pennsylvania Hospital if she had forgiven him for compelling her to submit to the remedies that had been employed for that purpose. "Forgive thee!" said she, "why I love the very ground thou walkest on."

If all the means that have been mentioned should prove ineffectual to establish a government over deranged patients, recourse should be had to certain modes of coercion. These will sometimes be necessary in order to prevent their destroying their clothes and the furniture of their cells, as well as to punish outrages upon their keepers and upon each other. The following means will generally be found sufficient for these purposes.

1. Confinement by means of a strait waistcoat, or of a chair which I have called a tranquillizer. - He submits to them both with less difficulty than to human force, and struggles less to disengage himself from them. The tranquillizer has several advantages over the strait waistcoat or mad shirt. - It opposes the impetus of the blood towards the brain, it lessens muscular action every where, it reduces the force and frequency of the pulse, it favours the application of cold water and ice to the head, and warm water to the feet, both of which I shall say presently are excellent remedies in this disease; it enables the physician to feel the pulse and to bleed without any trouble, or altering the erect position of the patient's body; and, lastly, it relieves him, by

means of a close stool, half filled with water, over which he constantly sits, from the foetor and filth of his alvine evacuations. [1]

2. Privation of their customary pleasant food.

3. Pouring cold water under the coat sleeve, so that it may descend into the arm pits, and down the trunk of the body.

4. The shower bath, continued for fifteen or twenty minutes. If all these modes of punishment should fail of their intended effects, it will be proper to resort to the fear of death. Mr. Higgins proved the efficacy of this fear, in completely subduing a certain Sarah T___, whose profane and indecent conversation and loud vociferations offended and disturbed the whole hospital. He had attempted in vain, by light punishments and threats, to put a stop to them. At length he went to her cell, from whence he conducted her, cursing and swearing as usual, to a large bathing tub, in which he placed her. "Now (said he) prepare for death. I will give you time enough to say your prayers, after which I intend to drown you, by plunging your head under this water." She immediately uttered a prayer, such as became a dying person. Upon discovering this sign of penitence, Mr. Higgins obtained from her a promise of amendment. From that time no profane or indecent language, nor noises of any kind, were heard in her cell.

By the proper application of these mild and terrifying modes of punishment, chains will seldom, and the whip never, be required to govern mad people. I except only from the use of the latter, those cases in which a sudden and unprovoked assault of their physicians or keepers may render a stroke or two of a whip, or of the hand, a necessary measure of self-defence.

To encourage us in the use of all the means that have been mentioned for subduing the tempers of mad people, and acquiring a complete government over them, I shall only add to the history I have given of their disease, that there is a predisposition in their minds to be acted upon by them, founded in their timidity. They are not only afraid of their keepers and attendants, but of one another. Some years ago a madman of the name of Hoops disturbed the whole village of Chester, in this state, by his conduct. A person more mad than himself came into the town. Hoops instantly ran from him, and took shelter in the court house while the court was sitting. There was an instance of the same timidity in a madman in our hospital, in the month of February 1810. In consequence of the house being unusually crowded with mad people, two men were confined in one cell. One of them, who, was very noisy, was instantly silenced by the rebukes of his less deranged companion. He even crept into a corner of the cell to avoid him.

The remedies for general mania come next under our consideration. In enumerating them, I shall adopt the same order that I followed in treating upon partial insanity, by mentioning,

I. Such as should be applied to the mind, through the medium of the body; and.

II. Such as should be applied to the body through the medium of the mind.

I. The first remedy under this head should be blood-letting.

This evacuation is indicated,

1. By all the facts and arguments formerly mentioned, in favour of this grade of madness being an arterial disease, of great morbid excitement or inflammation in the brain, particularly by the state of the pulse, and, when this is natural, by the state of the countenance, by wakefulness, and by a noisy and talkative disposition.

2. By the appetite being uninterrupted, and often unrestrained, whereby the blood-vessels become overcharged with blood.

3. By the importance and delicate structure of the brain, which forbid its bearing violent morbid action for a length of time, without undergoing permanent obstruction or disorganization. The danger from this cause is much increased by the wakefulness, hollowing, singing, and strong muscular exertions of persons in this state of madness.

4. By there being no outlet from the brain, in common with other viscera, to receive the usual results of disease or inflammation, particularly the discharge of serum from the blood-vessels.

5. By the accidental cures which have followed the loss of large quantities of blood. Many mad people, who have attempted to destroy themselves by cutting their throats, or otherwise opening large blood-vessels, have been cured by the profuse haemorrhages which have succeeded those acts. Of this, several instances have occurred within my knowledge.

6. By the morbid appearances of the blood which has been drawn for the cure of this form of madness. It is generally diseased beyond that grade in which it exhibits a buffy coat. Of 200 patients bled by Mr. Halsam, in the Bethlehem Hospital, the blood was sizy in but six cases, and from the cause that has been assigned. I have seen nearly all the morbid appearances of the blood which I have enumerated in my defence of blood-letting, and never a single instance in which it put on a natural appearance.

7. Blood-letting is indicated by the extraordinary success which has attended its artificial use in the United States, and particularly in the Pennsylvania Hospital.

In the use of bleeding in this state of madness, the following rules should be observed:

1. It should be copious on the first attack of the disease. From 20 to 40 ounces of blood may be taken at once, unless fainting be induced before that quantity be drawn. It will do most service if the patient be bled in a standing posture. The effects of this early and copious bleeding are wonderful in calming mad people. It often prevents the necessity of using any other remedy, and sometimes it cures in a few hours.

2. It should be continued not only while any of those states of morbid action in the pulse remain which require bleeding in other diseases, but in the absence of them all, provided great wakefulness, redness in the eyes, a ferocious countenance, and noisy and refractory behaviour continue, all of which

indicate a highly morbid state of the brain. We bleed in the same natural state of the pulse in the pneumonia notha. We do the same thing in a similar form of hepatitis.

The propriety of bleeding in this *mania notha,* if I may be allowed to use a term founded upon the unity of its cause (that is, congestion of blood without inflammation) with the causes of the above diseases of the lungs and liver, has often been demonstrated in the Pennsylvania Hospital. Its advantages, I well recollect, attracted the attention of the pupils of the hospital in the year 1805, in a more than ordinary manner, in the case of a man of the name of Pickins. His madness was recent, his skin was cool, and his pulse natural, but his eyes suffused with blood, and he was unable to sleep. I bled him copiously, after which his pulse became frequent and tense. I repeated the bleeding, and gave him several doses of purging physic, which cured him in a few days.

3. It should be more copious in phrenimania and synochomania, than in simple madness. Its liberal use is particularly indicated in the latter, when it is formed by the union of madness with pregnancy, or with the autumnal or puerperal fever, in all which the blood-vessels labour under disease in other parts of the body, as well as the brain.

4. It should be less copious in madness from drunkenness, than from any of its other causes, all the circumstances that call for it being equal. For the reasons for this caution, the reader will please to consult the defence of bloodletting, in the third volume of the author's Medical Inquiries and Observations.

5. It is indicated no less in the seventh and eighth forms of general mania, formerly described, than in those which preceded them. I think I once prevented suicide by it, in a young gentleman descended from a family in which several of its members had perished by their own hands,

6. The quantity of blood drawn should be greater than in any other organic disease. This is indicated not only by most of the reasons for bleeding formerly given, but by the strong and uncommon hold which the disease takes of the brain. Many circumstances prove this to be the case, but none more than its not being cured, and scarcely suspended, by the acute and painful disease of parturition, several instances of which have come under my notice. From among many cases of the successful issue of profuse bleeding in this form of madness, I shall select but two: the former was in Mr. T. H. of the state of New Jersey, a man of sixty-eight years of age, from whom I drew nearly 200 ounces of blood, between the 20th of December and the 14th of February in the year 1807: the latter was in Mr. D. T. of the state of New York, who lost about 470 ounces, by my order, by 47 bleedings, between the months of June 1810 and April 1811. Both these gentlemen were my private patients in the Pennsylvania Hospital. Were it necessary I could add to these cases several others, communicated to me by my pupils, particularly by Dr. Wallace, of Virginia, and Dr. Annan, of Maryland, in which a similar practice had been attended with the same success.

After all the symptoms which call for bloodletting have disappeared, we sometimes observe the disease to continue. In this case morbid excitement becomes insolated, but still so considerable as not to yield to purges or blisters. Here **cupping** is indicated. The cups should be applied to the temples, behind the ears, and to the nape of the neck. Leeches may be used for the same purpose, and to the same places. They may likewise be applied to the hemorrhoidal vessels with advantage, in persons who have been subject to the piles. The sympathy of the brain with these vessels is so intimate, that the disease yields as readily to the loss of blood from them, as from the parts that have been mentioned near the brain.

Arteriotomy performed upon the temporal artery, it is said, is more useful than venesection, or local bleeding with cups and leeches. I can say nothing in its favour from my own experience.

I have only to add to these remarks upon the use of cups and leeches, that they are not only useless, but often hurtful, if applied before the action of the pulse is reduced. By inducing debility in the blood-vessels of the brain, they invite morbid excitement to it from the blood-vessels of the trunk and extremities of the body, provided they retain a predominance, or even an equality of action with the blood-vessels of the brain.

3. **Solitude** is indispensably necessary in this state of madness. The passions become weak by the abstraction of company, and by refraining from conversation. For this reason visitors should be excluded from the cells and apartments of highly deranged people, and there are times in which the visits of a physician, and of the cell-keeper or nurse, should be as seldom and short as are consistent with the proper treatment and care of the patient.

4. **Darkness** should accompany solitude in the first stage of this disease. It invites to silence, and it induces a reduction of the pulse, by the abstraction of the stimulus of light, and by the influence of fear which is naturally connected with darkness. There are four cells in the Pennsylvania Hospital, so formed that it is possible to render them dark with but little trouble. I have seen the happiest effects from confining noisy patients in them.

5. An **erect** position of the body. There is a method of taming refractory horses in England, by first impounding them, as it is called, and then keeping them from lying down or sleeping, by thrusting sharp pointed nails into their bodies for two or three days and nights. The same advantages, I have no doubt, might be derived from keeping madmen in a standing posture, and awake, for four and twenty hours, but by different and more lenient means. Besides producing several of the effects of the tranquillizing chair, it would tend to reduce excitement, by the expenditure of excitability, from the constant exertion of the muscles which support the body. The debility thus induced in those muscles would attract morbid excitement from the brain, and thereby relieve the disease. That benefit would arise from preventing sleep, I infer from its salutary effects in preventing delirium, and from delirium being always increased by it in fevers of great morbid excitement.

6. **Low diet,** consisting wholly of vegetables, and those of the least nutritious nature. What would be the effect of fasting for two or three days in this state of madness? I am disposed to think favourably of it, from a fact communicated to me by a gentleman who resided twenty years in the interior parts of India He informed me that the wild elephants, when taken, are always tamed by depriving them of food, until they discover signs of great emaciation. They are then fed with mild aliment, and soon acquire their usual flesh, but without the least return of their ferocity. Fasting is calculated to act in two ways, in the cure of tonic madness; 1, by lessening the quantity of blood by the abstraction of aliment; and 2, by exciting the disease of hunger in the stomach to such a degree, as to enable it to predominate over the disease of the brain, and by that means attract it to a less vital part of the body. The effects of this severe remedy in curing inflammatory dropsy, render it still more probable that it might be employed, with advantage, in this disease of the brain. Against its use it may be said, that the ferocity of certain wild animals is increased by hunger; this is true, but ferocity is not derangement. It is possible it might exist for a little while, and be attended with symptoms totally different from those which take place in madness, and of a nature that would yield more easily to the power of medicine.

The drinks of a patient in this state of madness should be of the most simple kinds.

7. **Purging.** Cremor tartar, salts, senna, calomel and jalap, have all been employed for this purpose. Their use is indicated by the obstructions in the viscera, and torpor of the alimentary canal, which generally accompany this form of madness. There are cases in which the purges should be given daily, so as to excite an artificial diarrhoea. Nature, as I shall say presently, sometimes cures madness in this way. It is much in favour of this chronic mode of purging, that few persons are ever delirious in their last moments, who die of discharges from their bowels. In the mixture, which sometimes takes place, of mania with the synochus form of bilious fever, purging should be employed more freely than in simple madness. Calomel and jalap should be preferred for that purpose.

8. **Emetics** are spoken of very differently by authors. Some commend, while others condemn, them. When they have done harm, it must have been by giving them before, or after, the system was reduced below the emetic point. When given at that point, they have done good in many cases. I mentioned formerly their manner of operating, in treating of their efficacy in partial derangement.

9. **Nitre** has done the same service in this disease, that it has done in other diseases which affect the blood-vessels. Its efficacy is increased by such additions of tartarized antimony and calomel to it, as shall increase its disposition to act upon the bowels and skin.

10. **Blisters,** like emetics, have been considered as remedies of doubtful efficacy; but it is only because they have not been employed in the manner,

or at the precise time, that was necessary to obtain benefit from them. In a letter which I received in the year 1794, from Dr. Willis, senr. he informed me that he always applied them to the ankles in this disease, instead of the head or neck. He gave no reason for this practice, but it immediately suggested a principle to me, from which I have derived great advantages, not only in the treatment of madness, but of several other diseases. In the first stage of tonic, or violent, madness, the disease is intrenched, as it were, in the brain. - It must be loosened, or weakened, by depleting remedies, before it can be dislodged, or translated to another part of the body. When this has been effected, blisters easily attract it to the lower limbs, and thus often convey it at once out of the body. The same reasoning applies, with equal force, and the same practice with equal success, to all the violent diseases of the breast and bowels. The blisters do the same service, when applied to the wrists, and still more, when applied at the same time, or alternately, to both extremities. - After the complete reduction of the pulse, they may be applied with advantage to the neck and head.

11. **Cold,** in the form of air, water and ice. The cold air should be applied both partially and generally. To favour its partial action, the hair should be cut off, and shaved from every part of the head. Dr. Moreau, a French physician, has related a cure of madness performed by this simple remedy alone. How far the hair, by its sympathy with the brain, which it discovers by preternatural dryness in the forming state of many diseases, and by the alteration in its figure, colour, and quantity, from the influence of certain emotions and passions of the mind, may increase this disease, we know not; but we are certain, by cutting it off, we not only expose the head to a greater degree of cold, but we favour by it, at the same time, depletion from the brain, by means of insensible perspiration; for, however strange it may appear, there is a grade of action in the perspiring vessels , in which their discharges are increased by the sedative operation of cold.

Cold air, by its action upon the whole body, has likewise done service in this state of madness. I have heard of two instances, in which it was cured by the patients escaping from their keepers in the evening, and passing a night in the open air in the middle of winter. One of them relapsed; in the other the cure was permanent.

Cold water should be applied in like manner to the head, and the whole body. To the former it should be applied by means of cloths, or a bladder, to which ice, when it can be obtained, should be added; for the head, from its greater insensibility to cold than any other part of the body, feels, in but a feeble degree, the coldness of simple water. I have found this to be a more effectual, as well as a more delicate, mode of applying cold to the head, than by means of the clay cap, as advised by Dr. Cullen. The water, or ice, should be frequently renewed, and they should be continued for several days and nights. The signal for removing them should be, when they produce chilliness, and sobbing or weeping in the patient. The advantages of these cold applications to the head will be much increased, by placing the feet at the same time in warm water. The circulation is thereby more promptly equalized. The reader will find a striking instance of the efficacy of using cold and warm water in this manner to the two extremities, by my advice, in a case of mania published by Dr. Spence, of Dumfries, in Virginia, in Dr. Coxe's Medical Museum.

In order to derive benefit from the application of cold water to the whole body, it should be immersed in it for several hours, by which means we prevent the reaction of the system, and thus render the sedative effects of the water permanent. Pumping for an hour or two upon a patient acts in the same way; but as it has sometimes been employed in curing a fit of drunkenness, and may be considered as a punishment, rather than a remedy, immersion of the body should be preferred to it. The patience and insensibility of the system to cold, in this state of the system, is illustrated by a striking fact, mentioned by Dr. Currie in his Medical Reports. He tells us, a deranged young woman slept upon a cold floor during a whole night, so cold as to freeze water and milk upon her table, without suffering the least inconvenience from it.

11. **A salivation**. I mentioned the manner in which this remedy operated upon the brain, the bowels, and the mind, in treating of the cure of hypochondriac derangement. Too much cannot be said in its favour in general madness. I once advised it in a case of this disease from parturition, in which the patient conceived an aversion from the infant that had been the cause of her suffering. On the day she felt the mercury in her mouth, she asked for her infant, and pressed it to her bosom. From that time she rapidly recovered.

It is sometimes difficult to prevail upon patients in this state of madness, or even to compel them, to take mercury in any of the ways in which it is usually administered. In these cases I have succeeded, by sprinkling a few grains of calomel daily upon a piece of bread, and afterwards spreading over it a thin covering of butter.

12. The **Peruvian bark.** In all those cases in which mania is complicated with the intermitting fever, or with those prostrate states of fever in which bark is usually administered, this medicine may be given with advantage.

I have thus enumerated the principal remedies, which have been employed in reducing the preternatural excitement of the system which takes place in tonic madness. There are some others which have been employed for the same purpose, upon which I shall make a few remarks.

12. **Opium**. From an erroneous belief in the supposed sedative power of this medicine, it has been prescribed in this state of derangement, but I believe always with bad effects. When given in small doses, so as to prevent sleep, and by that means gradually to waste the excitability, or what Dr. Darwin calls the sensorial power of the system, it may be useful.

14. **Digitalis**. I have occasionally administered this medicine in tonic madness, but never with any radical or permanent success.

15. **Camphor** has been supposed to possess specific virtues in this state of madness. I have often prescribed it when a young practitioner, but without any obvious advantage. I should feel some hesitation in bearing a testimony against this, and the preceding medicine, had I not lately discovered that my experience of their inefficacy in this disease, accords with that of the ingenious Dr. Ferriar. They have both derived their credit in madness from their lessening the frequency of the pulse, in which, disease has very improperly been supposed to consist. But the frequency of a pulse may be lessened, without a reduction of its force, and even both may be effected by these medicines upon the pulse on the wrist, and yet irregular action in the blood vessels of the brain, which constitutes the disease, still continue, and until this be removed, they are calculated to do harm, by inducing obstructions in the brain, and thereby perpetuating the disease.

When madness arises from drunkenness, those medicines are safer and more useful, than when it arises from those causes which require copious blood-letting. In addition to them, volatile salts, bitters, and small quantities of ardent spirits, may be given with advantage, provided the system be first moderately reduced by the vise of depleting remedies.

I suspect many, and perhaps all, the cures that have been performed by opium, digitalis, and camphor, have been of madness from the intemperate use of strong drink. The disease in most of these cases partakes of the nature of a soap bubble. With all its apparent force, it is both feeble, and transient, and not only bears stimulants with safety, but sometimes requires them immediately after gentle evacuations of any kind.

16. **Hellebore** has been famed, for many centuries, as a specific for madness. It is generally admitted that it is useful, only, when it acts as a purge.

17. Dr. Gregory, senr. used to relate, in his lectures, a method of curing tonic madness, which was practised by a farmer in the neighbourhood of Aberdeen, in Scotland. It consisted in yoking a number of madmen in a plough, and compelling them, by fear or force, to plough his fields. This remedy acted, by reducing and expending the morbid excitement of the system. Refractory domestic animals are sometimes subdued in the same way; but experience has taught us that they may be tamed by more gentle means. Experience has proved, in like manner, that the system in tonic madness may be reduced by remedies that offer less violence to humanity, and that do not add to the affliction of the disease, by degrading the patient to a level with our domestic animals.

18. As soon as the disease shows signs of abatement, the patient should be relieved from his confinement, in order to partake of the benefits of fresh air and exercise. Swinging, riding in a carriage, and moderate walking, will be highly proper in this state of his disease. To these should be added,

19. The **shower bath**. This excellent remedy acts upon the head, by the stimulus arising from the weight and momentum of the water, and by the reaction of the blood-vessels after the sedative effects of the water are over. I

have seen very happy results from it. To do much service, it should be used two or three times a day.

20. The diet and drinks of the patient should now be of a cordial nature; and where obstinate wakefulness or restlessness attends, opium may be given at bed-time with safety and advantage.

21. When the disease affects the nervous and muscular systems, in common with the blood-vessels, with hysterical or convulsive symptoms; assafoetida, castor, and the oil of amber, should be given with all the remedies that have been mentioned.

II. We come next to mention the remedies that are proper to act upon the body through the medium of the mind.

1. The first remedy under this head is to divert the ruling passion or subject which occupies the mind, if it be *one,* and fix it upon some other. Nothing effectual can be done without great attention to this direction. The author has endeavoured to show, in an inquiry into the influence of physical causes upon morals, how much the passions may be made to neutralize and decompose each other, and thus to lessen their influence upon the body. History furnishes several examples of the truth of this remark. I mentioned formerly the effects of opposing the fear of shame to a false opinion in religion, in preventing suicide in the virgins of Miletus. Achilles was diverted by his mother Thetys from gratifying his revenge upon the body of Hector, by supplanting that baneful passion by the passion of love. Anger, and even rage, have often been opposed with success by terror and fear, and deliberate malice by a delicate stroke of wit. Where the mind is deranged upon *all* subjects, we should endeavour to fix it upon but *one.* In order to do this, it will be necessary to find out the favourite studies and amusements of our patients. The late Dr. Ash, Dr. Priestly informed me, was cured of derangement upon a variety of subjects, by seducing him to the study of mathematicks, of which he had been fond in early life. The distracted mind of the poet Cowper was composed, while he was employed in the single business of translating Homer; and I have heard of a woman who was cured of madness, by keeping her constantly employed for several days in playing cards, to which it was known she had always had a strong attachment. There are few persons so much deranged, as not to exhibit, for a half an hour or more, marks of correctness of mind, when drawn into conversation upon some subject not connected with their derangement. I admit that this diversion of the passions and understanding cannot be effected, where the *whole* mind, and all the passions, are under the influence of madness. Thus the virgins of Miletus could not have been cured by an appeal to the female sense of shame, had their moral faculties partaken of the disease of their other passions; nor could Dr. Ash have been cured of his intellectual derangement by the study of mathematicks, had he lost all his recollection of quantity and numbers.

2. A sudden sense of the **absurdity, folly,** or **cruelty** of certain actions, produced by conversation, has sometimes cured madness. The cure in this

case bears a resemblance to the sudden reduction of a dislocated bone. Some years ago a maniac made several attempts to set fire to our hospital. Upon being remonstrated with, by Mr. Coats, one of its managers he said, "I am a salamander;" "but recollect (said Mr. Coats) all the patients in the hospital are not salamanders;" that is true, said the maniac, and never afterwards attempted to burn the hospital. Many similar instances of a transient return of reason, and some of cures, by pertinent and well directed conversations, are to be met with in the records of medicine.

3. Madness has sometimes been cured by the influence of **place, time,** and **company,** upon the human mind. In favour of the benefits of association from place, I shall mention the following facts. Vansweiten relates a story of a cabinetmaker, who always recovered his reason as soon as he entered his work-shop. A certain Mrs. D___, of this city, formerly a patient of mine, on the 27th of March 1792, was suddenly seized with derangement on her way from market. She rambled for two hours up and down the city, and at length was conducted to her own house. The moment she looked around her, she recovered her reason, nor did she relapse afterwards. I have known one clergyman, and have heard of another, who were deranged at all times, except when they ascended the pulpit, in which place they discovered, in their prayers and sermons, all the usual marks of sound and correct minds. I once attended a judge, from a neighbouring state, who was rational and sensible upon the bench, but constantly insane when off it. *Time,* by its influence upon a deranged mind, sometimes produces healthy and regular associations of ideas and conduct. The late Rev. Dr.___, of Baltimore, was observed to be less deranged on Saturdays, than on any other day of the week, probably from that day being formerly devoted exclusively to retirement and study, in preparing for the exercises of the ensuing Sabbath. *Company* has a similar effect in restoring healthy and regular associations in the mind. It should always be of that kind which produced respect in former times. It will readily occur to the reader, that all these remedies, derived from association, will be proper only in the declining and moderate state of the disease.

4. Great care should be taken by a physician, to suit his conversation to the different and varying states of the minds of his patients in this disease. In its furious state, they should never be *contradicted,* however absurd their opinions arid assertions may be, nor should we deny their requests by our answers, when it is improper to grant them. In the second grade of this disease, we should *divert* them from the subjects upon which they are deranged, and introduce, as if it were accidentally, subjects of another, and of an agreeable, nature. When they are upon the recovery, we may *oppose* their opinions and incoherent tales by reasoning, contradiction, and even ridicule. I attended a lady some years ago in our hospital, in whom this practice succeeded to my wishes. In the first and raving state of her disease, she said the spirit of general Washington visited and conversed with her every night. I took no notice of this assertion, but prescribed only for the excited state of her pulse. After

this was reduced, I entered into conversation with her, and instantly obtruded a subject foreign to the nightly visits of the spirit of general Washington, whenever she mentioned it. One day, when she appeared rational upon all the subjects upon which we conversed, she lifted up the skirt of her silk gown, and said, "See what a present general Washington made me last night!" O! fie! said I, Madam, I thought you had more understanding than to suppose general Washington would leave his present abode, to bring a silk gown to any lady upon the face of the earth. She laughed at this rebuke, and never mentioned the name of general Washington to me afterwards, nor discovered any other mark of the remains of her disease.

From the history of this case, we see there are the same acquiescing, diverting, and opposing points in this grade of madness, that were mentioned in treating upon the cure of tristimania, and amenomania, all of which should be carefully attended to, in conversing with persons who are affected with it.

We see further from this case, that the cure of mental and bodily disease is to be effected by the same means. We first reduce the system, then create revulsive actions, and finally remove subsequent debility, or feeble morbid actions, by stimulating remedies. From the nature of the last of these remedies, the necessity of rescuing maniacal patients from solitude must be very obvious, in order to their producing a salutary effect. Indeed they should never be confined a day after they cease to be disposed to injure themselves or others.

5. The return of regularity and order in the operations of the mind will be much aided, by obliging mad people to read with an audible voice, to copy manuscripts, and to commit interesting passages from books to memory. By means of the first, their attention will be more intensely fixed upon one subject than by conversation. In this way only, they read when alone, and in this way only, they comprehend what they read. They revert in this respect to the state of childhood. - By copying manuscripts, the attention will be still more fixed to one subject, and abstracted from all others. I have witnessed the most salutary effects from it, particularly in a gentleman from New England, whose cure was completed by transcribing a volume of lectures for a student of medicine. Committing select passages from books to memory will be more useful than either of them, inasmuch as it requires greater efforts of mind to accomplish it. To facilitate this mode of exciting and regulating the faculties and operations of the mind, a few entertaining books of history, travels, and prints, should compose a part of the shop furniture of every public and private mad-house.

6. **Music** has been much commended in this state of madness. History records two cures of royal patients being affected by it. Dr. Cox mentions a striking instance of its power over the mind of a madman. It should be accommodated to the state of the disease. In that grade of it which is now under consideration, the tunes should be of a plaintive, that is, of a sedative nature.

7. **Terror** acts powerfully upon the body, through the medium of the mind, and should be employed in the cure of madness. I once advised gentle exercise upon horseback, in the case of a lady in Virginia who was deranged. In one of her excursions from home, her horse ran away with her. He was stopped after a while by a gate. The lady dismounted, and when her attendants came up to her, they found her, to their great surprise and joy, perfectly restored to her reason, nor has she had since the least sign of a return of her disease. A fall down a steep ridge cured a mania of twenty years continuance. Dr. Joseph Cox relates three cures of madness by nearly similar means. Dr. M. Smith, of Georgia, informed me, that a madman had been suddenly cured in Virginia, by the breaking of a rope, by which he had been let down into a well that was employed as a substitute for a bathing tub. He was nearly drowned before he was taken out. The cures in all these cases were effected, by the new actions induced in the brain by the powerful stimulant that has been mentioned. In the use of it, great care will be necessary to suit its force to the existing state of the system.

8. **Fear,** accompanied with **pain,** and a sense of **shame,** has sometimes cured this disease. Bartholin speaks in high terms of what he calls "flagellation" in certain diseases. I have heard of several instances of its efficacy in tonic madness. Two soldiers were cured by it in the American army, during the revolutionary war. A madman, who escaped from his keepers in Maryland, ran to one of his neighbours with an intention to kill him. His neighbour met him with a heavy whip, and beat him until he fell upon his knees, and implored him to spare his life. He rose from his knees in a sound state of mind, and had no symptom of his disease afterwards. In mentioning the cures performed by the whip, let it not be supposed that I am recommending it in this slate of madness. Fear, pain, and a sense of shame, may be excited in many other ways, that shall not leave upon the memory of the patient the distressing recollection, that he owes his recovery to such a degrading remedy.

9. How far artificial **grief** might be employed with advantage in this disease, I shall not determine, but I have heard of its having been suspended for several days, in a clergyman now in the Pennsylvania Hospital, by the death of one of his children; and of mania of five years standing, descending to manalgia, in a lady in New York, by hearing: of the death of her husband. It caused her to weep for several weeks. The disease in this case, which had been diffused through all her passions, was suddenly concentrated in but one of them, and in her understanding, from whence it gradually passed out of her system. If these facts should not be deemed a sufficient warrant to create artificial grief, they will show that relief may be expected, from communicating to persons affected with this grade of madness the intelligence of the death of their relations and friends.

10. Convalescents from derangement should be defended from the **terrifying** or **distressing noises** of patients in the raving state of this disease, by removing the latter to small lodges, remote from the hospital, or private

mad-houses, or by confining them in cells that are made with double walls, doors, and windows, so as to obstruct the passage of sound. A relapse has often been induced by the neglect of this caution.

[1] A chair such as has been described may be seen in the Pennsylvania Hospital, and an engraving of it in the test volume of Dr. Coxe's Medical Museum.

Chapter Seven - II. Of Manicula

This second grade of general madness, which I have called manicula, differs from mania, as chronic rheumatism differs from that which is acute, that is, in being accompanied with a more moderate degree of the same symptoms. The pulse is usually synochula, typhoid or typhus. It is in this state of madness that we discover that peculiar sensibility to cold, which is generally absent in its highest and lowest grades. Shakespeare, who saw this disease in common life, and out of the restraints and conveniences of a hospital, has very happily illustrated this symptom in the character of Edgar, whom he often makes to exclaim in, counterfeiting madness, "poor Tom's a cold." From the operations of fresh exciting causes, manicula now and then rises into mania, in which state it is sometimes cured, but it oftener descends in a few days or weeks to its chronic, or habitual form. It is now and then combined with typhus fever, in which state it has been called by Dr. Cullen typhomania. We see it occasionally in the last stage of the puerperal, the jail, and autumnal fever.

The **remedies** for this grade of madness should be the same in its inflammatory state as for mania, but of less force. In its typhoid and typhus states, they should be the same as in the declining state of mania, with the addition of garlic in substance or infusion, and the different preparations of iron. In the typhomania, the remedies should be combined with those usually employed in the treatment of typhus fever, particularly bark and opium. The latter is an invaluable medicine in such cases. The dose of it should be much larger than in common diseases of the same grade of action.

Chapter Eight - III. Of Manalgia

The symptoms of this third and last form of general madness are, taciturnity, downcast looks, a total neglect of dress and person, long nails and beard, dishevelled or matted hair, indifference to all surrounding objects, insensibility to heat and cold. A remarkable instance of insensibility to the latter occurred in a certain Thomas Perrin, who was admitted into the Pennsylvania Hospital, with manalgia, in March 1765, and who died there in September 1774, during all which time he ate and slept in the cupola of the hospital, and never, in the coldest weather of nine winters, came near to a fire. A fixed position of the body sometimes attends this form of madness. Of this there have been two remarkable instances in our hospital. In one of them, the patient sat with his body bent forward for three years, without moving, except when compelled by force, or the calls of nature. In the other, the patient occupied a spot in a ward, an entry, or in the hospital yard, where he appeared more like a statue than a man. Such was the torpor of his nervous system, that a degree of cold, so intense as to produce inflammation and gangrene upon his face and limbs, did not move him from the stand he had taken in the open air. The cause of this young man's insanity was as singular as its nature. It was induced by his father's selling a pleasant farm, upon the Delaware, in the neighbourhood of Philadelphia, on which he was born, and had passed his youth, and which he expected to inherit after the death of his father. The skin in manalgia is dry, cold, pale, yellow, brown, lived, and dark coloured, and now and then covered here and there with black spots. The eyes, when originally dark, acquire a light colour in this disease. I took notice formerly of the prevalence of this colour in the deranged patients in the Pennsylvania Hospital. It probably arises from the tendency of the system to dissolution, for we frequently see it in the last stage of pulmonary consumption, and it rarely fails to take place in old age. The appetite in manalgia is inordinate or weak, the bowels are costive, the urine is scanty in quantity, and there is sometimes a discharge or slabbering of saliva. This symptom with one other, was selected by David, when he counterfeited madness, in order to prevent the discovery of his person by the king of Gath, after his escape from the hands of Saul. "And he changed his behaviour before them (says the sacred historian) and feigned himself mad, and scrabbled upon the doors of the gate, and let his spittle fall down upon his beard." The discharge of saliva in this case appeared to be involuntary, and in this we perceive a distinguishing mark between manalgia and tonic madness, in the latter of which, I said formerly, the saliva is discharged with difficulty by spitting. The respiration is slow, the breath and perspiration have a peculiar and offensive smell, and the pulse is languid and frequent, but sometimes natural. Nebuchadnezzar seems to have been affected with this low grade of madness. He was said to resemble a beast, probably from the uncommon growth of his hair, beard, and nails.

A strong attachment to tobacco is common in the patients who have been previously in the habit of using it. They frequently ask strangers for it, or for a few cents to buy it.

These are the usual symptoms of manalgia in hospitals, but when persons who are affected with it possess their liberty, they rather seek for, than shun human society. They are often admitted by private families to pass nights in their kitchens, garrets, or barns. Sometimes they wander through neighbourhoods in the capacity of beggars. Shakspeare has described this state of derangement, very accurately, in the character of Edgar, in King Lear, when he makes him adopt the resolution of counterfeiting the character of a madman.

"I will (says Edgar) take the basest and poorest shape,
That ever penury, in contempt of man,
Brought near to beast. My face I'll grime with filth,
Blanket my loins, tie all my hair with knots,
And, with presented nakedness, outface
The winds, and persecutions of the sky:
And with this horrible object, from low farms,
Poor pelting villagers, sheep cotes, and mills,
Sometimes with lunatic bans, sometimes with prayers,
Enforce their charity."

There are some instances in which the moral faculties are impaired in manalgic patients, in which case they are mischievous and vicious, but they are more generally inoffensive, and disposed to be kind, and even useful, in hospitals and families. In some of them, the sense of Deity is not only unimpaired, but in an elevated state. The mad poet, Christopher Smart, often kneeled down and prayed in the streets of London, when he was permitted to leave his house, and he never suffered any of his visitors to leave him, without requesting them to pray with him.

A late poet has described this pious form of manalgia, in a young woman, very happily in the following lines:

"But her praise was still, to be
Where holy congregations bow.
Wrapt in wild transports, while they sang;
And when they pray'd, would bow her low."

Madness in this form sometimes continues for ten, fifteen, twenty, and even fifty years, when not accompanied with paroxysms, but it more generally terminates in death in a shorter time, and frequently by diseases, to be mentioned hereafter.

The equanimity of temper, together with the want of exercise, and the inordinate appetite, which generally accompany this disease, sometimes produce obesity. They had that effect, Dr. Johnson tells us, upon Mr. Smart. I have seen two instances of it in Philadelphia.

The **remedies** for **manalgia** should consist, like those under a former head, of such as act,

I. Upon the mind, through the medium of the body; and,

II. Upon the body, through the medium of the mind.

I. To the first head belong,

1. Cordial food and drinks. The former should be made savoury and grateful to the taste, and the stimulus from the pleasure imparted by it should be increased by its variety. The latter should consist of wine, cyder and malt liquors. Ardent spirits should be given with great caution, lest a destructive fondness should be acquired for them. There is least danger of this being the

case, when they are given in an undiluted state once or twice a week. I have seen the most beneficial effects from them, when administered in this manner. To patients in whom this form of madness has been induced by intemperance in drinking, they may be given daily, and in liberal quantities.

2. The warm bath. The water should be heated *above* the natural temperature of the body, in which state it acts powerfully upon the arterial system. I have once known it induce 150 strokes in the pulse in a minute, and excite the brain into delirium, in an experiment made upon himself by a student of medicine in the university of Pennsylvania. From the occasional effects of fevers, which act in a similar way upon the blood-vessels, I have been led to think highly of the remedy. An epidemic fever, many years ago, pervaded the cells of our hospital, which restored the greatest part of the maniacs to their reason. These accidental cures struck the late Dr. Bond so forcibly, that he attempted to excite a fever in several of his patients in manalgia afterwards, by sending them to the swamps of Gloucester county, near to the city, in the state of New Jersey. With what success I have never heard.

3. The **cold shower bath**. The impulse imparted to the head by the descent of the water upon it adds very much to its efficacy, and gives it great advantages over the plunging bath.

4. The **cold** shower bath, in succession to the **warm** bath. While I attended the Pennsylvania Hospital in the summer of 1785, I often employed these two remedies in the manner I have mentioned. I kept my torpid patient in the warm bath for an hour or two, and then led him, smoking with vapour, to the shower bath, which gave a most powerful shock to his system. It extorted cries and groans from persons that had been dumb for years. In one case it relieved, and in another, it restored reason to my patient; but from his being confined in a damp cell, he died some time after his recovery from his madness, of a pulmonary consumption.

5. Exciting an artificial diarrhoea. In the tonic state of madness, purging, I said formerly, acted as a depleting remedy. In manalgia it does good, by exciting a revulsive action or disease, in a less delicate part of the body than the brain. Nature, I said formerly, sometimes cures manalgia in this way. An instance of a cure from this cause occurred in our hospital some years ago, in a woman who had been deranged nine years. An acute dysentery cured it in a woman in Chester county, after it had continued two years. It may be excited by a laxative diet, or any gently opening medicine.

6. **A caustic** applied to the back of the neck, or between the shoulders, and kept open for months or years. This remedy acts by the permanent discharge it induces from the neighbourhood of the brain. Four patients have been cured of manalgia in our hospital, by abscesses in different parts of the body. One of them had passed a third of his life in the hospital. Dr. Johnson tells us, in his Lives of the Poets, that Dean Swift had a temporary return of his reason during the continuance of an abscess in his eye.

7. **A salivation**. I know it is difficult to excite this disease in the throat and mouth in manalgia, but the mercury, if given ineffectually for this purpose, will be useful as a general stimulant and tonic. It will moreover serve to remove visceral obstructions, which so generally succeed madness. Where it excites a salivation, it seems to recuscitate the mind. I have seen two instances in our hospital, in which a taciturnity of a year's continuance was removed by it. Speech was excited, in one of them, on the very day on which the mercury affected the mouth, and the use of reason followed in a few days afterwards.

8. **Exercise**. This should consist of swinging, seesaw, and an exercise discovered by Dr. Cox, which promises more than either of them, and that is, subjecting the patient to a rotatory motion, so as to give a centrifugal direction of the blood towards the brain. He tells us he has cured eight persons of torpid madness by this mode of exercise. I have contrived a machine for this purpose in our hospital, which produces the same effects upon the body which are mentioned by Dr. Cox. These are vertigo and nausea, and a general perspiration. I have called it a Gyrater. It would be more perfect, did it permit the head to be placed at a greater distance from us centre of motion. It produces great changes in the pulse. In one experiment made with it, it increased the pulse from 84 to 88 strokes in one minute, and to 120 in two minutes. It increased its fulness at the same time. In a second experiment made upon a manalgic patient, it increased the frequency of the pulse from 104 in two minutes to 150. In a third experiment it reduced the pulse from 108 in three minutes to 100, and lessened its force. In this patient, the pulse was preternaturally active before he entered the gyrater.

From the strong impression this mode of exercise makes upon the brain, there is reason to believe it will be a useful remedy in manalgia. A cheap contrivance, to answer all its purposes, might easily be made, by placing a patient upon a board moved at its centre upon a pivot, with his head towards one of its extremities, and then giving it a rotatory motion. The centrifugal force of the blood would exceed, in this way, that which it receives from the chair employed by Dr. Cox, or from the gyrater in the Pennsylvania Hospital. In addition to these exercises, pleasant amusements should be contrived for this class of mad people. If they are unhappy, these amusements will suspend their misery. If they are in a torpid state, a transient sense of pleasure will be excited by them, which may serve to remind them that the chain is still unbroken which united them with their fellow men.

9. **Labour** has several advantages over exercise, in being not only more stimulating, but more durable in its effects, whereby it is more calculated to arrest wrong habits of action, and to restore such as are regular and natural. It has been remarked, that the maniacs of the male sex in all hospitals, who assist in cutting wood, making fires, and digging in a garden, and the females who are employed in washing, ironing, and scrubbing floors, often recover, while persons, whose rank exempts them from performing such services,

languish away their lives within the walls of the hospital. In favour of the benefits of labour, in curing this disease, I shall select one from among many facts that might be mentioned. In the year 1801 I attended an English gentleman, soon after his arrival in America, who was afflicted with this grade of madness. My prescriptions relieved, but did not cure him. He returned to his family in Maryland, where, in the time of hay harvest, he was allured into a meadow, and prevailed upon to take a rake into his hands, and to assist in making hay. He worked for some time, and brought on thereby a profuse sweat, which soon carried off his disease. This account of his remedy and cure I received from himself, in a very sensible letter written a few weeks after his recovery. I have often wished, and lately advised, that the mad people in our hospital should be provided with the tools of a number of mechanical arts. Some of them should be laborious, and employ the body chiefly; others ingenious, and of a nature to exercise and divert the mind more than the body. None of them should be carried on by instruments, with which it would be easy for the maniacs to hurt themselves or others. For certain exploits of industry or skill, they should receive such rewards in food, or dress, as accord most with their inclinations, for few of them are capable of any higher or other gratification. The advantages of thus producing a current of new actions, both corporeal and mental, which should continue for weeks and months, and perhaps years, could not fail of being accompanied with great advantages. Some emolument might likewise be derived from their labour to their friends, or to the institution that supported them. What a different view would a number of mad people exhibit, all thus imitating the habits of rational industry, compared with the antic gestures, the rapid or sauntering walks, the listless attitudes, and the vociferous or muttering conversations they hold with themselves, with which they excite pity or horror in all who see them.

In both the exercises and labours of mad people, they should be as much separated from each other as possible. We are naturally imitative animals; and our minds are formed in a degree by ambient circumstances; for which reason mad people should associate and work only with persons of sound and healthy minds.

10. **Music** should not be omitted as a remedy in this state of madness. The tunes employed tor this purpose should be of the most invigorating nature.

11. **Great pain.** Mr. Stewart, the pedestrian traveller, informed me, that he once saw a transient interval of reason induced upon several idiots in Italy, by means of torture, inflicted from pious, but superstitious, motives, by some priests. - Dr. Cox mentions an instance of chronic madness being cured by trepanning, and of the same good effects being produced by accidental contusions of the head. It is probable they both acted only by inducing pain. The return of reason, which I shall say hereafter sometimes takes place in the last hours of life, is probably occasioned, in part, by the bodily pains which attend the passage out of life. Should this remedy be resorted to, it should be in-

duced by means that are not of a degrading nature, and which are calculated at the same time to excite some violent passion or emotion of the mind.

12. **Errhines.** These are suggested by the general absence of secretion in the nose in mad people, and by the relief which the discharge of a few drops of tears affords in tristimania. The insensibility of the nose to the stimulus of common snuff, from its habitual use by that class of patients, forbids us to expect any benefit from it, for which reason the sulphate of mercury, and the muriate of ammonia, mixed with a little flour, should be preferred for that purpose.

13. **Certain odours.** The dyer, formerly mentioned, informed me, that he had often observed the men that were employed in dying scarlet to be uncommonly cheerful, and sometimes to sing from morning till night. The odour which produces this effect is derived from a mixture of cochineal with a solution of tin in the nitric acid. The exhilaration produced by the fragrance of a flower garden in the spring of the year, and of the Spice Islands in the Indian Ocean, favours the idea still more, of exciting the brain by means of pleasant odours applied to the organ of smelling.

14. What would be the effect of loud and uncommon **sounds,** acting through the ears, upon the brain and mind in this disease? Menalgic patients, it has been observed, are much excited by the military music that sometimes passes by the Pennsylvania Hospital. It is still more in favour of loud sounds, or noises, in manalgia, that in the lowest stage of typhus fever, they have recalled departing life; and in asphixia, restored it from its apparent extinction in death.

15. Exciting certain stimulating **passions** and **emotions,** also the domestic **affections**. I mentioned several instances of the good effects of terror, in tristimania, and in tonic madness in its declining state. To be useful in manalgia, it should be often repeated. Of the good benefits of anger, I shall mention a striking instance. - Mr. Derborow, whose name was mentioned formerly, during his long confinement in our hospital, in a state of manalgia, became silent for several months. Many attempts were made to compel him to speak, but to no purpose. The late Dr. Thomas Bond at length contrived to force him to break his long and obstinate silence. It was the practice of Mr. Derborow to amuse himself occasionally during this time in drawing. One day the Doctor looked over his shoulder, and saw the picture of a flower under his pencil. "A very pretty cabbage," said the Doctor. "You are a fool and a liar," said Mr. Derborow, "it is a flower." From that time he continued to speak as usual. Reading aloud and incorrectly to patients in this situation has sometimes induced a transient feeling of uneasiness or irritation, which has unsealed their lips, and revived their former habits of conversation.

The advantages to be expected from exciting the domestic affections will appear from the following fact. A woman in our hospital was delivered, many years ago, of a fine child during her derangement, which was of a chronic and torpid nature. The affection which was suddenly awakened for this child, removed her disease for several days. The child was taken from her breast, lest it should contract the seeds of madness from her milk. Her disease immediately returned, and she is now, and probably always will be, an incurable tenant of our hospital.

There are several medicines which have been given in this disease, upon which I shall make a few remarks. These are,

16. Opium, iron, the datura stammonium, strong infusions of green tea and green coffee, garlic, valerian, the nitrous oxyd, and electricity.

I have administered all these medicines in this disease in the Pennsylvania Hospital, and some of them for several months, but never in a single instance with success, when given alone. Garlic now and then produced a temporary frequency and fulness in the pulse, and electricity has produced a transient excitement in the temper, but neither of them made a permanent impression upon the disease. Where a recovery has succeeded the use of any of those medicines, I have supposed the disease was cured by time, instances of which will be mentioned hereafter. In thus stating the inefficacy of the above medicines in manalgia, I would by no means reject them altogether. They may be given as auxiliaries to those more powerful and rational remedies which agitate the whole body and mind.

In the use of all our remedies for manalgia, an advantage will arise from prescribing them in succession and rotation, and in choosing certain seasons of the year, according to the habits of the patient, for their exhibition.

To encourage us to persevere for years in the use of remedies for this disease, or to wait for a cure from the hand of time, founded upon those spontaneous changes that are always going forward in the human body, I shall select two cases of recoveries from among many others, the one from the former, the other from the latter cause.

1. In the year 1795 a young man of the name of Donaldson, from York county, in Pennsylvania, was admitted into our hospital in the lowest state of manalgia. He had been in that situation between four and five years. He appeared to have no mind, and scarcely any locomotive powers. When placed at the head of a pair of stairs, he rolled to the bottom of it. By means of most of the remedies I have recommended, he was nearly cured. He acquired the use of his speech, knew his attendants, and called me by my name when I visited him. Unhappily, in his progress to a perfect cure he was attacked with a malignant fever, and died in the hospital on the fifth day of his disease.

2. The following account of a spontaneous recovery was communicated to me, many years ago, by Dr. A. Hunter, with his History of the Lunatic Asylum in York, in Great Britain.

"On the twenty-fifth of October, 1778, a seafaring person, about forty years of age, was recommended to the Lunatic Asylum for cure. - About two years before that time he had sustained a considerable loss by sea, which operated so violently upon his mind, as to deprive him, almost instantly, of all his reasoning faculties. In that state of insensibility he was received into the Asylum. During his abode there, he was never observed to express any desire for nourishment; and so great was his inattention to this particular, that for the first six weeks it was necessary to feed him in the manner of an infant. Food and medicines were equally indifferent to him. A servant undressed him at night, and dressed him in the morning; after which he was conducted to his seat in the common parlour, where he remained all day with his body bent, and his eyes fixed upon the ground. From all the circumstances of his behaviour, he did not appear to be capable of reflection. Every thing was indifferent to him; and from the fairest judgment that could be formed, he was considered by all about him as an animal converted *nearly* into a vegetable. In this state of insensibility he remained till the morning of Tuesday the fourteenth of May, 1783, when, upon entering the parlour, he saluted the recovering patients with a "Good morrow to you all." He then thanked the servants of the house, in the most affectionate manner, for their tenderness to him; of which, he said, he began to be sensible some weeks before, but had not till then the resolution to express his gratitude. A few days after this unexpected return to reason, he was permitted to write a letter to his wife, in which he expressed himself with decency and propriety. At this time he seemed to have a peculiar pleasure in the enjoyment of the open air, and in his walks conversed with freedom and serenity. Talking with him on what he felt during the suspension of reason, he said that his mind was *totally* lost; but that about two months before his return to himself, he began to have thoughts and sensations: these, however, only served to convey to him fears and apprehensions, especially in the night time. With regard to his medical treatment, I shall only observe, that the medicines usually prescribed for melancholic persons were, in his case, studiously avoided, and, instead of evacuants, cordials and a generous diet were constantly recommended. Had the natural powers been weakened, I am satisfied that the mind never would have regained her empire. During the remainder of his stay in the Asylum, he continued to behave himself with steadiness and propriety. He ate and drank moderately, and upon all occasions showed a gentle and benevolent disposition. Finding his mind sufficiently strong, he returned to his family on the twenty-eighth of May, 1783. Soon after this he was appointed to the command of a ship employed in the Baltic Trade, in which service he is at this time engaged."

I shall dismiss the history of all the different forms of madness, and of their respective remedies, by remarking that they do not always occur in the order in which they have been described. Partial and general madness sometimes precede and sometimes succeed each other. Manicula sometimes exists without mania, and both, without being succeeded by manalgia. There are instances in which manalgia has preceded mania, and manicula; and lastly, we now and then see them all combine, and alternate with each other. From this view of the successive and alternate changes of the different forms of madness into each other, we derive fresh proofs of the unity of its cause, and the necessity of renouncing all prescriptions for its names, and of constantly and closely watching the disease, in order to vary our remedies with its varying forms.

I shall now make a few remarks, which are alike applicable to all the forms of general madness.

1. Great regard should be had to cleanliness in the persons and apartments of mad people. This is indispensably necessary, not only for their comfort, but their cure. A deranged man, with a ragged dress, a dirty skin, long nails and beard, and uncombed hair, or with his dress and person in neat order, in a filthy room, loses his consciousness of his personal identity; and until this be restored, it is in vain to expect a return of the natural habits of his mind. A close stool, with a pan half filled with water, in order to suffocate the foetor of his evacuations, should be fixed in his room, with a cover, which should fall down of itself upon the stool after it is used.

2. Mad people should never be visited, nor even seen by their friends, and much less by strangers, without being accompanied by their physician, or by a person to whom he shall depute his power over them. The dread of being exposed, and gazed at in the cell of a hospital by an unthinking visitor, or an unfeeling mob, is one of the greatest calamities a man can anticipate in his tendency to madness. The apprehension of it was so distressing to a young gentleman in this city in a fit of low spirits, that he prevented it, by discharging the contents of a loaded musket through his brain. But there is another advantage from concealing the persons of mad people from the eye of visitors and the public. The disease is supposed to fix something of a repelling nature upon persons and families, and hence it is often concealed or denied. Now, by rendering the place in which mad people are confined, private — I had almost said sacred — members of families may be sent there without its being known. Nay, they will be sent there upon the first appearance of the disease, in order to *prevent* its being known, and the disease thereby be more frequently cured. This privacy would act with peculiar force upon the female sex. The obliquity and convulsions of the moral faculties, which sometimes take place in madness, would in this way never be known, or, if known, would be forgotten, or never divulged. To render a hospital still more agreeable, or less the object of aversion by the female sex, they should be carefully separated from the men, and they should be nursed only by women.

3. In the history of all the forms of general madness, it was remarked that they were all attended, now and then, with the cheerfulness of amenomania, but oftener with the distress of hypochondriasm. In the latter case, it will be necessary to use all the precautions to prevent suicide, that were recommended in treating upon that disease.

4. We should be careful to distinguish between a return of reason and a certain cunning, which enables mad people to talk and behave correctly for a short time, and thereby to deceive their attendants, so as to obtain a premature discharge from their place of confinement. To prevent the evils that

might arise from a mistake of this kind, they should be narrowly watched during their convalescence, nor should they be discharged, until their recovery had been confirmed by weeks of correct conversation and conduct. Three instances of suicide have occurred in patients soon after they left the Pennsylvania Hospital, and while they were receiving the congratulations of their friends upon their recovery. The disease, in these cases, was probably revived by two causes,

1. By means of association, from the sight of persons or objects that first excited it, or that were first connected with it; and,

2. By exchanging the large and noisy society of the hospital, for the comparative solitude and silence of a private family.

The madness of Dr. Zimmerman, which had been suspended for three months by travelling, returned on the day he entered his own house. To prevent this fatal or distressing recurrence of madness, it would be a good practice to send patients abroad, or to reside for some time among strangers, before they returned to their families. All the means of destroying themselves should, at the same time, be kept out of their way.

The recurrence of madness, after it has been cured, is no objection to the power of medicine over it. There are frequent returns of catarrh, pleurisy, and intermitting fever, after they have been cured, and yet we do not ascribe them to the uncertainty or imperfection of our science. Of twenty -five persons that were cured of madness, by Mr. Pinel, but two relapsed in the course of five years, which is probably much less than the relapses which occur from the other diseases that were mentioned.

I cannot conclude this part of the subject of these Inquiries, without lamenting the want of some person of prudence and intelligence in all public receptacles of mad people, who should live constantly with them, and have the exclusive direction of their minds. His business should be, to divert them from conversing upon all the subjects upon which they had been deranged, to tell them pleasant stories, to read to them select passages from entertaining books, and to oblige them to read to him; to superintend their labours of body and mind; to preside at the table at which they take their meals, to protect them from rudeness and insults from their keepers, to walk and ride with them, to partake with them in their amusements, and to regulate the nature and measure of their punishments. Such a person would do more good to mad people in one month, than the visits, or the accidental company, of the patient's friends would do in a year. But further. We naturally imitate the manners, and gradually acquire the temper of persons with whom we live, provided they are objects of our respect and affection. This has been observed in husbands and wives, who have lived long and happily together, and even in servants, who are strongly attached to their masters and mistresses. Similar effects might be expected from the constant presence of a person, such as has been described, with mad people, independently of his performing for them any of the services that have been mentioned. We render a limb that has been broken, and bent, straight, only by keeping it in one place by the pressure of splints and bandages. In like manner, by keeping the eyes and ears of mad people under the constant impressions of the countenance, gestures, and conversation of a man of a sound understanding, and correct conduct, we should create a pressure nearly as mechanical upon their minds, that could not fail of having a powerful influence, in conjunction with other remedies, in bringing their shattered and crooked thoughts into their original and natural order.

In reviewing the slender and inadequate means that have been employed for ameliorating the condition of mad people, we are led further to lament the slower progress of humanity in its efforts to relieve them, than any other class of the afflicted children of men. For many centuries they have been treated like criminals, or shunned like beasts of prey; or, if visited, it has been only for the purposes of inhuman curiosity and amusement. Even the ties of consanguinity have been dissolved by the walls of a mad house, and sons and brothers have sometimes languished or sauntered away their lives within them, without once hearing the accents of a kindred voice. Happily these times of cruelty to this class of our fellow-creatures, and insensibility to their sufferings, are now passing away. In Great Britain, a humane revolution, dictated by modern improvements in the science of the mind, as well as of medicine, has taken place in the receptacles of mad people, more especially in those that are of a private nature. A similar change has taken place in the Pennsylvania Hospital, under the direction of its present managers, in the condition of the deranged subjects of their care. The clanking of chains, and the noise of the whip, are no longer heard in their cells. They now taste of the blessings of air, and light and motion, in pleasant and shaded walks in summer, and in spacious entries, warmed by stoves in winter, in both of which the sexes are separated, and alike protected from the eye of the visitors of the hospital. Inconsequence of these advantages they have recovered the human figure, and, with it, their long forgotten relationship to their friends and the public. Much, however, remains yet to be done for their comfort and relief. To animate us in filling up the measure of kindness which has been solicited for them, let us recollect the greatness of its object. It is not to feed nor clothe the body, nor yet to cure one of its common diseases it is to restore the disjointed or debilitated faculties of the mind of a fellow-creature [1] to their natural order and offices, and to revive in him the knowledge of himself, his family, and his God.

But in performing this achievement of skill and humanity, we not only confer a positive good, but we remove a positive evil, which has no parallel in the list of human sufferings. If there were no other reason to believe this was the case, than the distress which takes place from a slight irregularity in the circulation of the blood in the brain, in a great majority of our dreams, it would be sufficient to render their assertion probable; but we have many proofs of its being strictly true. The tearing of clothes, so common in this disease, was one of the instituted signs of deep distress among the Jews, and it was so probably, from its being one of its natural signs among the nations of the East. The hollowing, stamping with the feet, and the rattling of chains, so generally practised by mad people, are all resorted to, in order to excite such counter-impressions upon their ears, as shall suspend or overcome, by their force, the anguish of their minds. They wound and mangle their bodies for the same purpose. Even in those solitary cases of general madness, which are accompanied with singing and laughter, there is good reason to believe the heart is depressed with sadness. Nor are the silence, and seeming apathy of manalgia, always signs of the absence of misery. The "willow weeps," says the poet, "but cannot feel; the torpid maniac feels, but cannot weep." In maintaining the general existence of misery in all the forms of derangement, I am supported, not only by the acts that have been mentioned, but by the authority of Shakespeare, in the following view of the images and feelings that usually harrow up the imaginations of mad people.

"Who gives any thing (says Edgar) to poor Tom,
Whom the foul fiend has led through fire,
And through flame, through ford, and whirlpool,
Over bog and quagmire, that hath laid
Knives under his pillow, and halters in his pew,
Set rats-bane by his porridge, made him to
Ride upon a bay trotting horse, over four-inch
Bridges, and to course his own shadow for a traitor."

And again, Lear, in a language still more expressive of suffering, complains,

------------------------ "I am bound
Upon a wheel of fire, that mine own tears
Do scald like molten lead."

It is no objection to the correctness of this description of the distress and horror which distract the minds of mad people, that they often have no recollection of them after their recovery. Happily for them! this is prevented, by derangement affecting the memory as well as the understanding. Even in those cases of manalgia in which the mind loses its sensibility to misery, and the subjects of it cease to be objects of our sympathy, they do not forfeit their claims to our good offices. Though insensible of mental pain, they are still sensible of kindness, and of corporeal pleasure. A pleasant look, a kind word, an orange, an apple, or even a flower, presented to them in an affectionate manner, are cordials and donations of inestimable value. With these transient and casual favours should be united savoury food. This is the more necessary to them, as their senses of smell and touch, and often of hearing, are so much impaired as to cease to afford them any pleasure. Perhaps their food is more enjoyed by them upon that account.

I shall now mention the signs of a favourable and unfavourable issue of madness, in all the forms of it which have been described.

The longer its remote and predisposing causes have acted upon the brain, and mind, the more dangerous the disease, and vice versa.

General madness, which succeeds tristimania, or that comes on gradually, is more difficult to cure, than that which comes on suddenly. Here we see its affinity to fever.

Madness, which arises from a hereditary predisposition, is said to be more difficult to cure, than that which follows a predisposition to it that has been acquired. It is certainly excited more easily, and is more apt to recur when cured, but in general, its paroxysms yield to medicine as readily as madness from an acquired predisposition.

Madness from corporeal causes is more easily cured than from such as are mental.

The younger the subject, the more easy the cure. Of 467 persons cured in Bethlehem Hospital, between the years 1784 and 1794, who were between 20 and 50 years of age, 200 of them were between 20 and 30.

It is rarely cured in old people. Mr. Halsam says, of 31 persons in advanced life, who were admitted into Bethlehem Hospital, but four were cured in the course of ten years.

Persons who have children are more difficult to cure than those who are childless.

It is more easily cured in women than in men. Mania yields more readily to medicine than manigula, or manalgia. An 100 patients in mania in its furious state, and the same number in its chronic state, were selected in the Bethlehem Hospital, in order to determine their relative danger and obstinacy. Of the former 62 were cured, and of the latter but twenty-seven.

A paroxysm of mania succeeding manicula, or manalgia, is favourable.

A fever succeeding bleeding is favourable. It shows a suffocated disease to be changed into a diffused one. A malignant fever, I remarked formerly, once cured a number of maniacs in our hospital.

Remissions and intermissions of violent mental excitement, are always favourable.

Lucid intervals in manicula and manalgia are likewise favourable. They show that torpor has not completely taken possession of the brain.

Abscesses in any part of the body are favourable. I formerly mentioned instances of recoveries which succeeded them.

A running from, or moisture in the nose, after it has been long dry, is favourable.

Warm and moist hands, after they have been long cold and dry, are favourable.

A cessation of burning in the feet is favourable.

General anasarca is favourable, provided it has been preceded by bleeding. It was followed by a recovery in two cases in the Pennsylvania Hospital in the year 1811.

The continuance of hysterical symptoms, or their revival, after being long absent, is always favourable. The latter shows the disease to be passing from its seat in the blood-vessels to the nerves.

A moderate degree of obesity occurring during a remission of the disease is favourable. A greater degree of it is unfavourable.

A return of one regular stool daily, and at an habitual hour, is favourable.

A diarrhoea, when moderate, is favourable.

Madness, from the common causes of fever, from parturition, and from strong drink, generally yield to the power of medicine.

Madness from lesions of the brain is seldom cured.

Madness which succeeds epilepsy, or that is alternated with it, is, I believe, always incurable,

Madness which succeeds head-ache, palsy, and fatuity, is generally incurable.

Madness from emotions of the mind, such as anger, joy and terror, is more easily cured than when it arises from the passions. From the former causes it comes on suddenly, from the latter gradually.

Madness is difficult to cure, when it arises from the revival of an old and dormant passion, excited by association, especially when that passion is love or grief. It is remarkable, that the love which causes madness does not revive with its cure.

Gaiety, timidity, and good humour, are favourable. Ill-temper is unfavourable.

Weeping is favourable, when the disease has been preceded by hypochondriasm. It shows it to be changing into the less dangerous and distressing disease of hysteria.

Pensiveness and taciturnity often accompany and succeed a recovery from this disease. This is elegantly described in Orlando Furioso, after his recovery from madness induced by the unfaithfulness of his beloved Angelica.

Slow recoveries are most favourable.

A discharge of blood from the hemorrhoidal vessels, and the return of the menses, where they have been obstructed, are always favourable.

In three cases of madness that have occurred during pregnancy, within my knowledge, parturition did not cure, nor even mitigate them.

A return of spelling correctly, after it had been suspended, is favourable; so is a return of delicacy, more especially in the female sex.

The return of an habitual disease or appetite, shows an abatement of the violence of madness and is always favourable. The return of an habitual employment or of any of the habits of the understanding or the affections, that had been suspended, is still more favourable. I shall mention instances of each of them.

Sir George Baker declared the king of Great Britain to be convalescent from his first attack of madness, as soon as he heard him speak with a rapidity that had always been natural to him, and which he had lost during his insanity.

I attended a young man of the name of Wilkinson, in the Pennsylvania Hospital, in whom a habit of stammering was suspended during his derangement, but which returned as soon as he began to mend.

The return of diseases that are painful, such as head-ache, the rheumatism, the piles, or cough, also of tremors, and cutaneous eruptions, is still more favourable than the two cases of disease that have been mentioned.

A revival of an appetite for gingerbread, in a young man in our hospital, who had been fond of it when in health, was soon afterwards followed by his complete recovery.

A young lady in the neighbourhood of Philadelphia, who had been my patient for several weeks in an attack of madness from a fever, was observed by her family to call for her pen, ink, and common-place book, upon a Sunday. She had been in the practice of copying select pieces of poetry into it, for many years, upon that day of the week. At this time she discovered none of the common signs of the return of reason by her conduct or conversation. Trifling as this incident appeared, I encouraged her parents to expect from it a favourable change in her disease. It took place as I expected and she recovered perfectly in the course of a few weeks.

A female patient of mine, who had acquired pious habits when a child, practised them with great regularity during her derangement. Her recovery was marked by the gradual neglect of her devotion, and by a return of the gay and dissipated practices of her middle life.

A Mrs. D___, whom I supposed, for several months, had recovered from madness, under my care, said to me one day, in passing by her in our hospital, upon my asking her how she was, "that she was perfectly well, and that she was sure this was the case, for that she had at last ceased to hate me."

A similar instance of a perfect recovery succeeding the revival of domestic respect and affection occurred in a Miss H. L. who was confined in our hospital in the year 1800. For several weeks she discovered every mark of a sound mind, except one. She hated her father. On a certain day she acknowledged, with pleasure, a return of her filial attachment and affection for him; soon after she was discharged cured.

Spontaneous recoveries now and then occur, after the disease has continued 18 and 20 years. A recovery after the former period has lately taken place in a German farmer, in the county of Montgomery, in this state.

Maniacal patients sometimes die of its tonic or acute state, but in its chronic forms they more commonly die of some one of the following diseases.

1. Atrophy. Dr. Greding says 68 out of 100 patients die of this wasting disease.

2. Pulmonary consumption. It is remarkable that this disease does not so often suspend madness, as madness does pulmonary consumption.

3. Dropsy, particularly hydrothorax and anasarca, where they have not been preceded by bleeding. The latter disease aided madness in putting an end to the miserable life of Mr. Cowper.

4. A single convulsive fit, epilepsy, palsy, and apoplexy.

5. Fevers.

6. The disease induced by fasting.

It has been remarked, that patients who have long been confined in mad houses sometimes lose their hearing, but seldom their sight. I remarked formerly, that the ears are oftener affected with false perceptions than the eyes, in mad people; and from the nature of the disease which produces those false perceptions, it is easy to conceive that the sense of hearing must sooner perish than the sense of sight.

Most of mad people discover a greater or less degree of reason in the last days or hours of their lives. Cervantes therefore discovers both observation and judgment, in bringing Don Quixote to his senses just before he dies. Thus the sun, after a cloudy day, sometimes darts a few splendid rays across the earth just before he descends below the horizon. I have ascribed this resuscitation of reason in the paroxysm of death to the diseased blood-vessels relieving themselves by an effusion of water in the ventricles of the brain, or to the remains of the excitement of the system, awakened by fever, or pain, taking refuge in the mind.

[1] The following short extract, taken down by Mr. Coats, from the constant conversation of a young man of a good education, and respectable connections, now deranged in the Pennsylvania Hospital, will exhibit an affecting specimen of this disjointed state of the mind, and of the incoherence of its operations. "No man can serve two masters. I am king Philip of Macedonia, lawful son of Mary queen of Scots, born in Philadelphia. I have been happy enough ever since I have seen general Washington with a silk handkerchief in High-street. Money commands sublunary things, and makes the mare go; it will buy salt mackerel, made of ten-penny nails. Enjoyment is the happiness of virtue. Yesterday cannot be recalled. I can only walk in the night-time, when I can eat pudding enough. I shall be eight years old to-morrow. They say R. W. is in partnership with J. W. I believe they are about as good as people in common — not better, only on certain occasions, when, for instance, a man wants to buy chincopins, and to import salt to feed pigs. Tanned leather was imported first by lawyers., Morality with virtue is like vice not corrected. L. B. came into your house and stole a coffee-pot in the twenty-fourth year of his majesty's reign. Plumb-pudding and Irish potatoes make a very good dinner. Nothing in man is comprehensible to it. Born in Philadelphia. Our forefathers were better to us than our children, because they were chosen for their honesty, truth, virtue and innocence. The queen's broad R. originated from a British forty-two pounder, which makes two large a report for me. I have no more to say. I am thankful I am no worse this season, and that I am sound in mind and memory, and could steer a ship to sea, but am afraid of the thiller. ****** ****** son of Mary queen of Scots. Born in Philadelphia. Born in Philadelphia. King of Macedonia."

Chapter Nine - Of Demence, or Dissociation

Related to intellectual madness is that disease of the mind, which has received from Mr. Pinel the name of demence. The subjects of it in Scotland are said to "have a bee in their bonnets." In the United States, we say they are "flighty," or "hair-brained," and, sometimes, a "little cracked." I have preferred naming it, from its principal symptom, **dissociation**. It consists not in false perceptions, like the worst grade of madness, but of an association of unrelated perceptions, or ideas, from the inability of the mind to perform the operations of judgment and reason. The perceptions are generally excited by sensible objects; but ideas, collected together without order, frequently constitute a paroxysm of the disease. It is always accompanied with great volubility of speech, or with bodily gestures, performed with a kind of convulsive rapidity. We rarely meet with this disease in hospitals; but there is scarcely a city, a village, or a country place, that does not furnish one or more instances of it. Persons who are afflicted with it are good tempered and quarrelsome, malicious and kind, generous and miserly, all in the course of the same day. In a word, the mind in this disease may be considered as floating in a balloon, and at the mercy of every object and thought that acts upon it. It is constant in some people, but it occurs more frequently in paroxysms, and is sometimes succeeded by low spirits. The celebrated Lavater was afflicted with it; and although he wrote with order, yet his conversation was a mass of unconnected ideas, accompanied with bodily gestures, which indicated a degree of madness. I shall insert an account of a visit paid to him at Zurich by the Rev. Dr. Hunter, an English clergyman, in which he exemplified the state of mind I wish to describe.

"I was detained," says he, "the whole morning by the strange, wild, eccentric Lavater, in various conversations. When once he is set a going, there is no such thing as stopping him till he runs himself out of breath. He starts from subject to subject, flies from book to book, from picture to picture; measures your nose, your eye, your mouth, with a pair of compasses; pours forth a torrent of physiognomy upon you; drags you, for a proof of his dogma, to a dozen of closets, and unfolds ten thousand drawings; but will not let you open your lips to propose a difficulty; crams a solution down your throat, before you have uttered half a syllable of your objection.

He is as meagre as the picture of famine; his nose and chin almost meet. I read him in my turn, and found little difficulty in discovering, amidst great genius, unaffected piety, unbounded benevolence, and moderate learning, much caprice and unsteadiness; a mind at once aspiring by nature, and grovelling through necessity; an endless turn to speculation and project: in a word, a clever, flighty, good natured, necessitous man."

I said formerly, that hysteria consisted in mobility of the nervous and muscular system. Dissociation seems to be occasioned by a similar mobility of that part of the brain which is the seat of the mind.

The remedies for it, when it is attended with great excitement, as it generally is, should be, bleeding, low diet, purges, and all the other remedies for reducing morbid excitement in the brain, recommended formerly for the cure of intellectual madness.

When the disease is periodical, bark, and other tonics, should be given in its intervals.

Chapter Ten - On Derangement in the Will

Two opinions have divided philosophers and divines, upon the subject of the operations of the will. It has been supposed, by one sect of each of them, to act freely; and by the others to act from necessity, and only in consequence of the stimulus of motives upon it. Both these opinions are supported by an equal weight of arguments; and however incomprehensible the union of two such opposite qualities may appear in the same function, both opinions appear to be alike true.

The will is affected by disease in two ways.

I. When it acts without a motive, by a kind of involuntary power. Exactly the same thing takes place in this disease of the will, that occurs when the arm or foot is moved convulsively without an act of the will, and even in spite of it. The understanding, in this convulsed state of the will, is in a sound state, and all its operations are performed in a regular manner. When the will becomes the involuntary vehicle of vicious actions, through the instrumentality of the passions, I have called it **moral derangement**. For a more particular account of this moral disease in the will, the reader is again referred to a printed lecture delivered by the author, in the university of Pennsylvania, in November 1810, upon the Study of Medical Jurisprudence, in which the morbid operations of the will are confined to two acts, viz. murder and theft. I have selected those two symptoms of this disease (for they are not vices) from its other morbid effects, in order to rescue persons affected with them from the arm of the law, and to render them the subjects of the kind and lenient hand of medicine. But there are several other ways, in which this disease in the will discovers itself, that are not cognizable by law. I shall describe but two of them. These are, **lying** and **drinking**.

1. There are many instances of persons of sound understandings, and some of uncommon talents, who are affected with this **lying** disease in the will. It differs from exculpative, fraudulent and malicious lying", in being influenced by none of the motives of any of them. Persons thus diseased cannot speak the truth upon any subject, nor tell the same story twice in the same way, nor describe any thing as it has appeared to other people. Their falsehoods are seldom calculated to injure any body but themselves, being for the most part of an hyberbolical or boasting nature, but now and then they are of a mischievous nature, and injurious to the characters and property of others. That it is a corporeal disease, I infer from its sometimes appearing in mad people,

who are remarkable for veracity in the healthy states of their minds, several instances of which I have known in the Pennsylvania Hospital. Persons affected with this disease are often amiable in their tempers and manners, and sometimes benevolent and charitable in their dispositions.

Lying, as a vice, is said to be incurable. The same thing may be said of it as a disease, when it appears in adult life. It is generally the result of a defective education. It is voluntary in childhood, and becomes involuntary, like certain muscular actions, from habit. Its only **remedy**, is, bodily pain, inflicted by the rod, or confinement, or abstinence from food; for children are incapable of being permanently influenced by appeals to reason, natural affection, gratitude, or even a sense of shame.

2. The use of strong drink is at first the effect of free agency. From habit it takes place from necessity. That this is the case, I infer from persons who are inordinately devoted to the use of ardent spirits being irreclaimable, by all the considerations which domestic obligations, friendship, reputation, property, and sometimes even by those which religion and the love of life, can suggest to them. An instance of insensibility to the last, in an habitual drunkard, occurred some years ago in Philadelphia. When strongly urged, by one of his friends, to leave off drinking, he said, "Were a keg of rum in one corner of a room, and were a cannon constantly discharging balls between me and it, I could not refrain from passing before that cannon, in order to get at the rum."

The **remedies** for this disease have hitherto been religious and moral, and they have sometimes cured it. They would probably have been more successful, had they been combined with such as are of a physical nature. For an account of several of them, the reader is referred to the first volume of the author's Medical Inquiries and Observations. To that account of physical remedies I shall add one more, and that is, the establishment of a hospital in every city and town in the United States, for the exclusive reception of hard drinkers. They are as much objects of public humanity and charity, as mad people. They are indeed more hurtful to society, than most of the deranged patients of a common hospital would be, if they were set at liberty. Who can calculate the extensive influence of a drunken husband or wife upon the property and morals of their families, and of the waste of the former, and corruption of the latter, upon the order and happiness of society? Let it not be said, that confining such persons in a hospital would be an infringement upon personal liberty, incompatible with the freedom of our governments. We do not use this argument when we confine a thief in a jail, and yet, taking the aggregate evil of the greater number of drunkards than thieves into consideration, and the greater evils which the influence of their immoral example and conduct introduce into society than stealing, it must be obvious, that the safety and prosperity of a community will be more promoted by confining them, than a common thief. To prevent injustice or oppression, no person should be sent to the contemplated hospital, or **sober house**, without being examined and committed by a court, consisting of a physician, and two or three magistrates, or commissioners appointed for that purpose. If the patient possess property, it should be put into the hands of trustees, to take care of it. Within this house the patient should be debarred the use of ardent spirits, and drink only, for a while, such substitutes for them, as a physician should direct. Tobacco, one of the provocatives of intemperance in drinking, should likewise be gradually abstracted from them. Their food should be simple, but for a while moderately cordial. They should be employed in their former respective occupations, for their own, or for the public benefit, and all the religious, moral, and physical remedies, to which I have referred, should be employed at the same time, for the complete and radical cure of their disease.

2. Besides the disease in the will, which has been described, it is subject to such a degree of debility and torpor, as to lose all sensibility to the stimulus of motives, and to become incapable of acting either freely, or from necessity. In this respect it resembles a paralytic limb. We sometimes say of persons who are governed by their friends, or a favourite, that "they have no will of their own." This is strictly true. If left to themselves, they would neither buy nor sell, nor transact any kind of business. They *will*, and prefer nothing, and they do nothing, but what is closely connected with their animal existence. It is from the habitual want of exercise in the will in slaves, that it is so apt to acquire this paralytic state; and it is because we are deprived of its co-operation with our medicines in a desire of life, that we are less successful in curing their diseases under equal circumstances, than the diseases of freemen. Animal magnetism, Mr. Brisset informed me, performed many cures of light diseases upon the white people in the West Indies, but not a single slave was benefitted by it, and probably from the cause that has been mentioned.

I have never been consulted in this disease of the will, but I have no doubt stimulating and tonic remedies, preceded by depletion, would be useful in it. Persons afflicted with this disorder of the mind should be placed in situations, in which they will be compelled to use their wills, in order to escape some great and pressing evil. A palsy of the limbs has been cured by the cry of fire, and a dread of being burned. Why should not a palsy of the will be cured in a similar way?

Chapter Eleven - Of Derangement in the Principle of Faith, or the Believing Faculty

As this faculty has not yet found its way into our systems of physiology, I shall briefly remark, that I mean by it that principle in the mind, by which we believe in the evidence of the senses, of reason, and of human testimony. It is as much a native faculty as memory or imagination. The objects of human testimony are extensive and important. St. Paul alludes to them in the following passage of the eleventh chapter of his Epistle to the Hebrews. "Through faith we understand that the worlds were framed by the word of God, so that things which are seen were not made of things which do appear." The greatest part of all we believe of history, geography, and public events, and all that we believe of our relation to our parents, brothers and sisters, by the ties of consanguinity, are derived from it. Happily for us! its operations are involuntary in its sound state. Happily for us, likewise! a source of knowledge, so necessary to individual comfort and social existence, has not been made dependent upon our senses, nor left to the slow inductions of reason. The world could not exist in its present circumstances without it. It is no objection to its necessity and usefulness, that we are sometimes deceived by it. The same objection applies with equal force to our senses and reason, as sources of knowledge.

Persons affected with this disease in the principle of faith, as far as relates to human testimony, believe and report every thing they hear. They are incapable of comparing dates and circumstances, and tell stories of the most improbable and incongruous nature. Sometimes they propagate stories that are probable, but false; and thus deceive their friends and the public. There is scarcely a village or city, that does not contain one or more persons affected with this disease. Horace describes a man of that character in Rome, of the name of Apella. The predisposition of such persons to believe what is neither true, nor probable, is often sported with by their acquaintances, by which means their stories often gain a currency through whole communities.

It is probable the confinement of persons afflicted with this malady, immediately after they hear any thing new, might cure them. Perhaps ridicule might assist this remedy. I think I once saw it effectual in an old quidnunc during the revolutionary war.

This faculty of the mind is subject to disorder as well as to disease; that is, to an inability to believe things that are supported by all the evidence that usually enforces belief. Mr. Burke has described the conduct of persons affected with this disorder in the following words: "They believe nothing that they do not see, or hear, or measure by a twelve inch rule." An Indian once expressed the state of mind in which this torpor in the principle of faith takes place, by saying, when a truth was proposed to his belief, "that it would not believe for him." This incredulity is not confined to human testimony. It extends to the evidence of reason, and (it has been said) of the senses. The followers of Dr. Berkley either felt, or affected, the last grade of this disorder in the principle of faith. That it is often affected, I infer from persons who deny their belief in the utility of medicine, as practised by regular bred physicians, believing implicitly in quacks; also from persons who refuse to admit human testimony in favour of the truths of the Christian religion, believing in all the events of profane history; and, lastly, from persons who contradict the evidence of their senses in favour of matter, being as much afraid of bodily pain from material or sensible causes as other people.

The remedy for this palsy of the believing faculty, should consist in proposing propositions of the most simple nature to the mind, and, after gaining the assent to them, to rise to propositions of a more difficult nature. The powers of oratory sometimes awaken the torpor of the principle of faith. This was evinced, in a remarkable manner, in the speech which King Agrippa made to St. Paul, after he had heard his eloquent oration in favour of Christianity; "almost thou persuadest me to be a Christian." Perhaps great bodily pain would have the same, or a greater, effect in curing this disorder of the mind. It has often cured paralytic affections of the body, and of other faculties of the mind.

Sometimes a strong passion, or emotion, by pre-occupying the mind, prevents the exercise of belief. Thus we read, that the disciples of our Saviour could not believe the news of his resurrection "for joys." In such cases the predominating passion, or emotion, should be abstracted, or weakened, before an appeal is made to the principle of faith.

Chapter Twelve - Of Derangement in the Memory

This disease is attended with the following grades:

1. There is an oblivion of names, and vocables of all kinds.

2. There is an oblivion of names and vocables, and a substitution of a word no ways related to them. Thus I knew a gentleman, afflicted with this disease, who, in calling for a knife, asked for a bushel of wheat.

3. There is an oblivion of the names of substances in a vernacular language, and a facility of calling them by their proper names in a dead, or foreign language. Of this Wepfer relates three instances. They were all Germans, and yet they called the objects around them only by Latin names. Dr. Johnson, when dying, forgot the words of the Lord's prayer in English, but attempted to repeat them in Latin. Delirious persons, from this disease in the memory often address their physicians in Latin, or in a foreign language.

4. There is an oblivion of all foreign and acquired languages, and a recollection only of a vernacular language. Dr. Scandella, an ingenious Italian, who visited this country a few years ago, was master of the Italian, French and English languages. In the beginning of the yellow fever, which terminated his life, in the city of New York, in the autumn of 1798, he spoke English only; in the middle of his disease, he spoke French only; but on the day of his death, he spoke only in the language of his native country.

5. There is an oblivion of the *sound* of words, but not of the letters which compose them. I have heard of a clergyman in Newbury Port, who, in conversing with his neighbours, made it a practice to spell every word that he employed to convey his ideas to them.

6. There is an oblivion of the mode of spelling the most familiar words. I once met with it as a premonitory symptom of palsy. It occurs in old people, and extends to an inability, in some instances, to remember any more of their

names than their initial letters. I once saw a will subscribed in this manner, by a man in the eightieth year of his age, who, during his life, always wrote a neat and legible hand.

7. There is an oblivion of the qualities or numbers of the most familiar objects. I know a man in this city, who has never been able to remember the difference between a jug and a pitcher; and I know a physician, who for many years could not recollect that the umbilical cord consisted of two arteries and one vein, without associating the former with the double a in the last syllable of the name of Dr. Boerhaave.

There appears to be something like a palsy in the memory *quoad* these specific objects.

8. There is an oblivion of events, time and place, with a perfect recollection of persons and names. This is the case with the Rev. Dr. Magaw, formerly minister of St. Paul's church in this city. This disease in his memory was induced by a paralytic affection.

9. There is an oblivion of names and ideas, but not of numbers. We had a citizen of Philadelphia, many years ago, who, in consequence of a slight paralytic disease, forgot the names of all his friends, but could designate them correctly by mentioning their ages, with which he had previously made himself acquainted.

10. However strange it may appear, it has been remarked, that there is sometimes an oblivion of the most *recent,* the most *important,* and the most *interesting* events. Of this I could mention several instances that have come within my own knowledge. One of them occurred to Dr. Priestly. I have ascribed the oblivion of such events, to the memory being over stimulated from an undue effort to retain them. Something similar to it occurs in the inability of lovers to dream of each other.

The objects of knowledge either *perish,* or *sleep,* only in the mind. In the latter case, they are revived by means to be mentioned presently.

Wepfer takes notice of the following symptoms occurring with the loss or suspension of memory.

A sense of pain or heaviness in the forehead, a disposition to rub it with the hand, a formication, that is, a sense of something creeping up the left arm, and the fingers of both hands, a disposition to weep, and an involuntary flow of urine.

The causes of the weakness and loss of memory are corporeal and mental. To the first belong,

1. Intemperance in eating. Suetonius tells us the Roman emperor Claudius lost his memory so entirely from this cause, that he not only forgot the names and persons to whom he wished to speak, but even what he wished to say to them.

2. Intemperance in drinking. It was from the effect of strong drink, in weakening or destroying the memory, that an old Spanish law refused to

admit any person to be a witness in court that had been convicted of drunkenness.

3. Excess in venery.

4. Fevers, particularly such as are of a malignant nature, or that affect the brain. The Rev. William Tennent, formerly the pastor of a Presbyterian church at Freehold, in New Jersey, forgot every thing he had learned, even the letters of the alphabet, in consequence of an attack of a fever when he was about eighteen years of age.

5. Vertigo, epilepsy, palsy, and apoplexy.

6. Drying up an issue. Lesions of the brain.

7. The use of snuff. It was induced by this cause in sir John Pringle.

II. The mental causes are,

1. Grief. I once met with a woman, who had recently lost her husband and several children, who told me she forgot, at times, even her own name.

2. Terror. Artemidorus, a celebrated grammarian, was so terrified with the sight of a crocodile, that he immediately lost all the knowledge that he had treasured up in his memory in the course of his life.

3. Oppressing the memory in early life with words and studies disproportioned to its strength. The Latin and Greek languages, and the premature application of the mind to mathematics, I believe, have weakened or destroyed not only memory, but even intellect, in many young minds.

4. The undue exercise of the memory upon any one subject often weakens it upon all others. The famous African calculator Thomas Fuller, of Virginia, whose memory was exercised exclusively upon numbers, had so little recollection of faces, that he was unable to recognise the persons who had spent hours in conversing with him, and listening to his calculations, the next day after he saw them. Overcharging the memory with words has the same effect. A celebrated player in London, his son informed me, lost the recollection of the names of all his children, from this cause.

5. Neglecting to exercise the memory.

6. Cessation from study. Sir Isaac Newton forgot the contents of his "Principia" by ceasing to exercise his mind in study.

The famous Mr. Hude had spent several years in close application to conic sections. Leibnitz, in returning from his travels called to see him, and expected to have been highly entertained by conversing with him upon the subject of his studies. "Here," said Mr. Hude, sighing, "look over this manuscript. I have forgotten everything in it since I became burgomaster of Amsterdam."

The remedies for this disease are corporeal and mental.

To the First, or corporeal remedies, belong,

1. Abstracting all its exciting causes. Sir John Pringle's memory was restored, in a great degree, by leaving off the use of snuff.

2. Depleting remedies, if plethora attend, and the pulse be tense or oppressed. These should be, bleeding, purges, and low diet. After the reduction of the system, the remedies should be,

3. Blisters. Wepfer speaks in high terms of their efficacy, when applied to the elbows and calves of the legs, in this disease.

4. Issues in the arms.

5. Errhines.

6. Certain aromatic medicines. Etmuller says, when a young man, he greatly improved his memory by swallowing three or four cubebs every day. The cardamom seeds are said to have the same effect. Lavender and rosemary, or cloves, may be substituted for both of them.

7 The cold bath and cold weather. Milton's memory was always improved by the latter.

8. **Exercise.** Mr. Pope commends a trotting horse above all things in order to excite dormant ideas. It is from the motion excited in the brain, by means of a fever, that persons in that disease, often recollect events and speak languages, which appeared to have perished in their memories. The late Mr. Frederic A. Muhlenberg informed me that his father, who was for many years minister of the Lutheran church in Philadelphia, in visiting the old Swedes who inhabited the Southern district of the city upon their death beds, was much struck in hearing some of them pray in the Swedish language, who he was sure had not spoken it for 50 or 60 years before, and who had probably entirely forgotten it. It was revived by the stimulus of the fever in their brains which attended the close of their lives. The Rev. Dr. Muhlenberg of Lancaster has furnished me with a fact from his own observation, similar to that which was communicated to me by his brother, in the following extract of a letter which I lately received from him. "That people generally pray in their last hours in their native language is a fact which I have found true, in innumerable cases, amongst my German hearers, although hardly one word of German was spoken by them in common life and in days of health." Dr. Hutchinson, in his Biographia Medica, relates an anecdote of a physician of the name of Connor, who had renounced the principles of the church of Rome in early life, who, in the delirium of a fever which preceded his death, prayed only in the forms of that church. His fever had excited those forms, while those of the protestant religion which he had embraced were obliterated, by the same fever, from his mind.

In some cases, *time* performs a cure of the loss of memory. This oftenest occurs, when it has been induced by a fever. I have known one instance of it, and have heard of several others. One of the latter was in the Rt. v. Mr. Tennent, whose name was just now mentioned, who standing one day, at the feet of his master, suddenly threw down his grammar, and called for one of the Latin classics, which he had begun to read previously to the attack of his fever. At that instant all that he had ever learned before, revived in his mind.

The fever which deprived him of his memory was attended with apparent death for two or three days.

II. The mental remedies for the loss, or decay, of memory should be,

1. Frequently repeating what we wish to remember. The benefits of repetition are strikingly illustrated in the history of a printer in London, who, after working seven years in composing the bible, was able to repeat every chapter and verse in it by memory. We see the advantages of this mode of strengthening the memory, in persons who repeat questions or whole sentences that are proposed to them, before they can answer them. The door of the mind in such people requires two knocks before it can be opened, one by the person who asks, the other by the person who answers the questions; or, to speak more simply, the mind requires a double impression from words, before it is able to convert them into thoughts.

2. Calling in the aid of two or more of the senses, to assist in the retention of knowledge. We seldom forget what we have handled, or tasted, as well as seen or heard. It is for this reason that physicians who are educated in an apothecary's shop, never forget the sensible qualities or doses of medicines. The eyes assist the ears, and the ears the eyes. We are seldom satisfied in hearing a newspaper read; hence, when it is thrown down, we take it up, and convey to our minds, through the medium of our own eyes, the facts we have just before heard. Children and the vulgar, whose memories are alike weak, are unable to retain what they read, unless they receive it at the same time through their eyes and ears; hence the practice by both of them of reading when alone, with an audible voice. In some cases they are unable to remember even their own thoughts, without rendering them audible; hence we so often hear them talking to themselves. We observe the same thing in the low and chronic state of madness, and in part from the same cause. Where the eyes and ears cannot both be employed in acquiring knowledge, the use of the ears should be preferred. Julius Caesar says the reason why the ancient Druids did not commit their instructions to writing was, that their pupils might, by receiving them through their ears, more easily acquire, and more durably retain, them in their memories. The ear is less apt to be distracted than the eye by the obtrusion of surrounding objects, the one being more constant than the other. The mind moreover is more concentrated in hearing than in seeing. The truth of all these remarks is confirmed, by few of the sayings or songs learned by the ear only, and in the nursery, being ever forgotten.

3. The memory is restored and strengthened by means of association. The principal circumstances which influence this operation of die mind are, time, place, pleasure, pain, sounds, words, letters, habit and interest.

4. Filling the mind with that kind of knowledge only, which is supposed, or admitted, to be true. The errors and falsehoods which are crowded into the memories of boys, in our modern systems of education, are calculated ever

afterwards to weaken their retentive powers to such subjects as are true, and of a useful and practical nature.

5. The memory is improved by using it. Its low state among savages is occasioned by the small number of objects upon which they exercise it.

6. The memory is aided in hearing, and after reading, by shutting the eyes. In this way Mr. Woodfall received and retained the speeches of the members of the British parliament until he committed them to paper, after which he published and forgot them.

7. Ideas, and even words, that have been forgotten, are often recalled by conversation upon subjects that are related to them. This is effected by some incidental word, or idea, awakening by association the word, or idea, we wish to revive in our minds.

8. Dr. Van Rohr, a Danish physician, who visited this city in the year 1793, informed me that he could at any time excite the remembrance of words, by committing two or three lines of poetry to memory.

9. Singing aids the memory in acquiring a knowledge of words, and of the ideas connected with them. A song is always learned sooner than the same number of words not set to music. Virgil seems to have understood this perfectly, Hence he says,

--------------------"Saepe ego longas,
Cantando puerum, memini me
Condere."

10. Reading, or repeating what we wish to commit to memory, the last thing we do before we go to bed.

11. Learning a number of technical or arbitrary terms, and associating ideas with them. The rules for making syllogisms are taught in our systems of logic in this way. Dr. Grey's Memoria Technica may be read, with advantage, for much useful knowledge under this head.

Chapter Thirteen - Of Fatuity

This affection of the mind consists in a total absence of understanding and memory. It has different grades, from the lowest degree of manalgia, down to that which discovers itself in a vacuity of the eye and countenance, in silence or garrulity, slobbering, lolling of the tongue, and ludicrous gestures of the head and limbs.

It differs further, in being accompanied with activity in the will, or a total paralysis of it, and with active passions, or the total absence of them. The passions which most commonly appear in idiots are, anger, fear, and love. They moreover sometimes feel an inordinate degree of the sexual appetite, and are generally great feeders. Lastly, they are innocent, or extremely vicious.

Fatuity, or idiotism, is,

1. Congenial. In these cases the skull is less, and inferior in height to the skulls of maniacs, and there is a great disproportion between the face and head, the former being much larger than the latter. The bones of the head are preternaturally thick. This is the case we are told with the Cretins. Dr. Fodere, who has written an interesting account of them, says they have no knowledge of their parents, nor are they able to feed themselves until they are eight or ten years of age. All their senses are torpid. The venereal appetite exists in them with great force, and they gratify it after puberty by the practice of onanism. They are generally inoffensive, but now and then very mischievous. There is a case of congenial idiotism in a boy at Kensington, in the neighbourhood of this city, in which the powers of the body and mind are in a still lower state than in the Cretins. He was born on the 5th of August 1792, and is at this time unable to walk or speak. He has the head of a man, but all the parts of his body below it resemble those of a child of two or three years old, particularly his genitals and his pulse; the latter beats from 90 to 120 strokes in a minute. He has shed his teeth twice, and now exhibits a third set, in three distinct rows in his upper jaw. With all this furniture for mastication, he is unable to chew his food, and all that he takes of a solid nature is first chewed for him by his sister. His ears are very large. He cries when hungry and in pain, but oftener laughs for hours, and sometimes for whole nights together, and so loud as to disturb the sleep of his family. He discovers mind in but three things, viz. in an affection for his mother and sister, and in a love for a dog, and for money. His father sometimes comes home from his work in a state of intoxication, at which time he abuses his mother and sister. During this time he appears pensive, and refuses to eat any thing. He discovers distress when his dog is out of his sight, or his place in the family occupied by the dog of any of the neighbours. Of his love of money the following is a striking proof. I threw apiece of silver into his lap. He instantly laughed, and showed other signs of pleasure. I found upon inquiry that he was fond of gingerbread, and that he had just memory enough to associate the pleasure of eating it with the sight of the means of procuring it.

Fatuity is induced by all the causes which bring on mania, particularly by chronic fevers. It sometimes succeeds protracted manalgia. In complete fatuity, every part of the brain is torpid or paralytic, but where it exists with any of the passions we have mentioned, it is accompanied with partial diseased action in the brain.

3. Fatuity is induced by old age, in consequence of the brain becoming so torpid, and insensible, as to be unable to transmit impressions made upon it to the mind. It is partial; or general, according to the greater or less extent of the palsy of the brain.

Fatuity, whether a partial disease, or a disorder has been cured,

1. By another disease. The author has mentioned, in his Introductory Lecture upon the Study of Medical Jurisprudence, a curious instance of a young

woman, who was an idiot from her childhood, and continued so until her 35th year, at which time she was affected with pulmonary consumption. The impetus of the blood in the hectic fever of this disease, acting upon her brain, awakened her long dormant mind, and produced in her such marks of reason, that she astonished all her attendants by her conversation.

2. It has been cured by accidents, such as burns, and falls, and particularly when they affect the head. Dr. Haller relates a case of this kind. Dr. Nicholas Robinson mentions another, in which the cure was affected by a fall from a horse. After the disease induced by this fall ceased, the fatuity returned.

3. Time has sometimes cured fatuity. This has frequently been observed in that form of it which succeeds a chronic fever.

4. From the accidental effects of the remedies that have been enumerated, it is reasonable to expect, that powerful stimulants, which act alike upon the whole body and the brain, might be useful in fatuity. These remedies should be the same that were recommended formerly for the cure of manalgia. That form of fatuity, which sometimes follows a fever, generally yields to the most lenient of these remedies.

In order to assist all the remedies that have been mentioned, it will be useful, as soon as our patients begin to discover any marks of the revival of mind, to oblige them to apply their eye to some simple and entertaining book. They will much sooner acquire ideas in this way, than by our conversing with them, in consequence of the longer impressions of words upon the eyes than upon the ears, when they are pronounced in the ordinary rapid manner of common conversation. Dull boys are sometimes by this means ni.de scholars, and, on the contrary, boys of active minds are sometimes made dull by it. The forcible impressions of words in the latter case overstimulates the mind. Such boys learn more easily and rapidly by oral instruction.

Fatuity from old age cannot be cured, but it may be prevented, by employing the mind constantly in reading and conversation, in the evening of life. Dr. Johnson ascribes the fatuity of Dean Swift to two causes; 1, to a resolution he made in his youth, that he would never wear, spectacles, from the want of which he was unable to read in the decline of life; and, 2, to his avarice, which led him to abscond from visitors, or to deny himself to company, by which means he deprived himself of the only two methods by which new ideas arc acquired, or old ones renovated. His mind from these causes languished from the want of exercise, and gradually collapsed into idiotism, in which state he spent the close of his life in a hospital founded by himself for persons afflicted with the same disorder; of which he finally died.

Country people, who have no relish for books, when they lose the ability to work, or of going abroad, from age, or weakness, are very apt to become fatuitous, especially as they are too often deserted in their old age by the younger branches of their families, in consequence of which their minds become torpid, from the want of society and conversation. Fatuity is more rare in cities than in country places, only because society and conversation can be had in them upon more easy terms; and it is less common among women than men, only because they seldom survive their ability to work, and because their employments are of such a nature, as to admit of their being carried on by their fire sides, and in a sedentary posture.

The illustrious Dr. Franklin exhibited a striking instance of the influence of reading, writing, and conversation, in prolonging a sound and active state of all the faculties of his mind. In his eighty-fourth year he discovered no one mark, in any of them, of the weakness or decay usually observed in the minds of persons at that advanced period of life.

I cannot dismiss this subject without remarking, that the moral faculties, when properly regulated and directed, never partake of the decay of the intellectual faculties in old age, even in persons of uncultivated minds. It would seem as if they were thus placed beyond the influence, not only of time, but often of diseases and accidents, from their exercises being so indispensably necessary to our happiness, more especially in the evening of life.

The Rev. Dr. Magaw, I said formerly, had lost, with his memory for events, his consciousness of place and time, by a paralytic disease, and yet in this situation he retained, for several years, so high a sense of religious obligation, that he performed his devotions morning and evening, and at his meals, with as much regularity and correctness, as ever he did in the most vigorous and healthy state of his mind.

There is a state of fatuity, related to that which has been described, in which there exists, with great feebleness of mind, a species of low wit and cunning, accompanied at times with mimickry. Shakespeare has described this grade of idiotism, in his character of the fool, in the tragedy of King Lear. Such persons were formerly in demand at courts, as jesters, in order to dissipate, by their buffoonery, the ennui which is created by a superfluity of the enjoyments of life.

It is possible this mental disease might be relieved by the same remedies that have been recommended for common fatuity.

Chapter Fourteen - Of Dreaming, Incubus, or Night Mare, and Somnambulism

To enumerate all the phenomena of dreams, and to attempt an explanation of their proximate cause, would require a previous account of the theory of sleep, and this would render it necessary to introduce several phisiological principles, all of which would he foreign to the practical objects of this work; for which reason I shall barely remark, that dreaming is the effect of unsound or imperfect sleep. That this is the case is obvious, from its being uncommon among persons who labour, and sleep soundly afterwards, and from its causes to be mentioned presently. It is always induced by morbid or irregular action in the blood-vessels of the brain, and hence it is accompanied with the same erroneous *train,* or the same *incoherence* of thought, which takes place in delirium. This is so much the case, that a dream may be considered as a transient paroxysm of delirium, and delirium as a permanent dream. It differs from madness in not being attended with muscular action.

As dreams are generally accompanied with distress, and are often the premonitory signs of acute diseases, their cure is an important object of the science of medicine. Their remote cause are an increase, or diminution, of stimuli upon the brain.

I. The increased stimuli are corporeal, and mental.

1. The corporeal stimuli are, an excessive quantity of aliments or drinks, or of both, of an offensive quality to the stomach, a position of the head not habitual to the patient, cold, heat, noises, a tight collar or wrist-bands, a fever, opium, a full bladder, inclination to go to stool, and, lastly, light. It is from the stimulus of the last cause, that we dream most after day-break in the morning.

2. The mental stimuli are, all disquieting passions, difficult studies begun at bed-time, and an undue weight of business.

II. Dreams are induced by the diminution of habitual stimuli, such as customary food, drinks, exercise, labour, studies, and business. They are sometimes terrifying, or distressing, and not only detract from the happiness of life, but, when neglected, become the cause of more serious diseases in the brain. The remedies for them, when they are induced by an increase of stimuli, whether corporeal or mental, should be

1. Bleeding, or gentle purges, and low diet. The famous pedestrian traveller, Mr. Stewart, informed me that he never dreamed, when he lived exclusively upon vegetable food.

2. Exercise, or labour, which reduces excitement, and wastes excitability down to the point of natural and sound sleep. Persons who work hard during the day, seldom dream.

3. Avoiding all its remote and exciting causes, more especially such of them as act upon the mind in the evening.

4. When dreaming arises from a diminution of customary stimuli, a light supper, a draught of porter, a glass of wine, or a dose of opium, generally prevent them. Habitual noises, when suspended, should be restored.

Of the Incubus, or Night Mare

This disease is induced by a stagnation of the blood in the brain, lungs, or heart. It occurs when sleep is more profound than natural. Its remote causes are the same as of dreams. To these may be added sleeping upon the back, by which means the blood is disposed to stagnate in the places above mentioned, from an excess or diminution of the force that moves it. Persons who go to bed in good health, and are found dead in their beds in the morning, it is supposed, generally die of this disease.

Its remedies should be the same as for dreams, with the additional one of sleeping alternately on each side.

Of Somnambulism

I shall introduce my remarks upon this disease, by copying Dr. Hartley's correct and perspicuous account of its cause, in his "Observations upon Man."

"Those who walk and talk in their sleep (says the doctor) have evidently the nerves of the muscles concerned so free, as that vibrations [or nervous influence] can descend from the internal parts of the brain, the peculiar residence of ideas, into them. At the same time, the brain itself is so oppressed, that they have scarce any memory. Persons who read inattentively, that is, see and speak almost without remembering; also those who labour under such a morbid loss of memory, as that though they see, hear, speak and act, *pro ne nata,* from moment to moment, yet forget all immediately, somewhat resemble the persons who walk and talk in their sleep."

Dreaming, I have said, is a transient paroxysm of delirium. Somnambulism is nothing but a higher grade of the same disease. It is a transient paroxysm of madness. Like madness it is accompanied with muscular action, with incoherent, or coherent conduct, and with that complete oblivion of both, which takes place in the worst grade of madness. Coherence of conduct discovers itself, in persons who are affected with it undertaking, or resuming, certain habitual exercises or employments. Thus we read of the scholar resuming his studies, the poet his pen, and the artisan his labours, while under its influence, with their usual industry, taste and correctness. It extended still further in the late Dr. Blacklock, of Edinburgh, who rose from his bed, to which he had retired at an early hour, came into the room where his family was assembled, conversed with them, and afterwards entertained them with a pleasant song, without any of them suspecting he was asleep, and without his retaining, after he awoke, the least recollection of what he had done.

Persons who are affected with this disease sometimes appear pale, and covered with profuse sweats.

Its **remedies** should be the same as for dreaming, when it arises from an increase of corporeal or mental stimuli. I have read an account of two cures being performed, by placing a tub of water in the bedroom of patients who were afflicted with it.

Chapter Fifteen - Of Illusions

By this term I mean that disease, in which false perceptions take place in the ears and eyes in the waking state, from a morbid affection of the brain, or of the sense which is the seat of the illusion. It may be considered as a waking dream. Persons affected with it fancy they hear voices, or see objects that do not exist. These false perceptions are said, by superstitious people, to be premonitions of death. They sometimes indicate either the forming state, or the actual existence of disease, which being seated most commonly in a highly vital part of the body, that is the brain, now and then ends in death, and thus administers support to superstition. They depend, like false perception in madness, upon motion being excited in a part of the ear or the eye, which does not vibrate with the impression made upon it, but communicates it to a pan upon which the impression of the noise heard, or of the person seen, was formerly made, and hence the one becomes audible, and the other visible.

The deception, when made upon the ears, consists most commonly in hearing our own names, and for this obvious reason; we are accustomed to hear them pronounced more frequently than any other words, and hence the part of the ear, which vibrates with the sound of our names, moves more promptly, from habit, than any other part of it. For the same reason the deception, when made upon the eyes, consists in seeing our own persons, or the persons of our intimate friends, whether living or dead, oftener than any other people. The part upon the retina, from which those images are reflected, move more promptly, from habit, than any other of that part of the organ of vision.

The voice which is supposed to be heard, and the objects which are supposed to be seen, arc never heard nor seen by two persons, even when they are close to each other. This proves them both to be the effect of disease in the single person who hears, or sees, the supposed voice or object. I am aware that this explanation of illusions may be applied to invalidate the accounts that are given in the Old and New Testaments of the supernatural voices and objects, that were heard or seen by individuals, particularly by Daniel, Elisha, and St. Paul; but they should no more have that effect, than the cures of diseases that are performed by natural means should invalidate the accounts that are given in those books, of the same diseases being cured in a miraculous manner. But, admitting the voices or objects that were heard or seen, by the prophets and apostle above mentioned, to have been produced by a change in the natural actions of the brain, or of the organs of hearing or seeing, that change, considering its design, was no less supernatural, than if the voices or objects supposed to have been heard, or seen, had been real. It is remarkable, that in all those cases, where miracles were necessary to establish a divine commission, or a new doctrine, every circumstance connected with them was distinctly heard, or seen, not by an individual only, but by two or three, and sometimes by several hundred witnesses, in all of whom it is scarcely possible for an illusion to have existed at the same time from natural causes.

The remedies for illusions should be, bleeding, purges, and low diet, when the pulse indicates undue excitement in the arterial system. A certain Mr. Nicolai, a member of the academy of sciences in Berlin, was much relieved of this disease by the application of leeches to the hemorrhoidal vessels.

In a reduced state of the system, the remedies should be, cordial diet and tonic medicines. Mr. Nicolai heard the voices of his friends only when he was alone, and in a state of inaction. This fact suggests the advantages of company and exercise, as additional remedies in this disease.

Chapter Sixteen - Of Reverie or Absence of Mind

This disease is induced by two causes,

1. By the stimulus of ideas of absent subjects being so powerful, as to destroy the perception of present objects; and,

2. By a torpor of mind so great, as not to feel the impressions of surrounding objects upon the senses. It is an inferior or feeble grade of catalepsy.

It is more common from the latter than the former cause. It is no objection to this assertion, that it sometimes occurs in scholars, and in men celebrated for their great literary attainments. A capacity for acquiring knowledge is a cheap endowment, and differs widely from that capacity, which enables a man not only to acquire knowledge from books, but to create it by observation and reflection, and to apply it to the useful purposes of life. The following account of a clergyman who died a few years ago in England, extracted from a late periodical work, will serve to exhibit the nature and extent of this intellectual disease, from the latter cause that was mentioned.

"Mr. George Harvest, minister of Thames Ditton, was one of the most absent men of his time; he was a lover of good eating, almost to gluttony; and was further remarkable as a great fisherman; very negligent in his dress, and a believer in ghosts. In his youth he was contracted to a daughter of the bishop of London; but on his wedding day, being gudgeon fishing, he overstaid the canonical hour; and the lady, justly offended at his neglect, broke off the match. He had at that time an estate of 300*l.* per annum, but, from inattention and absence, suffered his servants to run him in debt so much, that it was soon spent. It is said, that his maid frequently gave bails to her friends and fellow servants to the neighbourhood; and persuaded her master that the noise he heard was the effect of wind.

In the latter part of his life no one would lend, or let him, a horse, as he frequently lost his beast from under him, or at least out of his hands, it being his practice to dismount and lead his horse, putting the bridle under his arm, which the horse sometimes shook off, and sometimes it was taken off by the boys, and the parson seen drawing his bridle after him.

Sometimes he would purchase a penny-worth of shrimps, and put them in his waistcoat pocket, among tobacco, worms, gentles for fishing, and other trumpery: these he often carried about him till they stunk so as to make his presence almost insufferable, I once saw such a melange turned out of his pocket by the dowager lady Pembroke. With all these peculiarities, he was a man of some classical learning, and a deep metaphysician, though generally reckoned a little crack'd.

Such was his absence and distraction, that he frequently used to forget the prayer days, and to walk into his church with his gun, to see what could have assembled the people there.

In company he never put the bottle round, but always filled when it stood opposite to him; so that he very often took half a dozen glasses running.

That he alone was drunk, and the rest of the company sober, is not, therefore, to be wondered at.

One day Mr. Harvest, being in a punt on the river Thames with Mr. Ostow, began to read a beautiful passage in some Greek author, and, throwing himself backwards in an ecstasy, fell into the water, whence he was with difficulty fished out.

Once being to preach before the clergy at the visitation, he had three sermons in his pocket: some wags got possession of them, mixed the leaves, and sewed them all up as one: Mr. Harvest began his sermon, and soon lost the thread of his discourse, and got confused; but nevertheless continued, till he had preached out first all the churchwardens, and next the clergy; who thought he was taken mad."

It is possible moderate depletion, succeeded by constant and noisy company, might product in the mind a predominance of impressions from present objects, over those of the ideas of absent subjects. Stimulants, particularly such as act upon the brain and nervous system, would probably be useful, when the disorder arises from torpor of mind, or insensibility of the senses.

Chapter Seventeen - Of Derangement of the Passions

The passions have been divided into two great classes, 1, such as are intended to impel us to real, or supposed good; and, 2, such as are intended to defend us from real, or supposed evil. The former are objects of desire, the latter of aversion. Those of them which are most subject to derangement, or to an unreasonable and morbid excess, are, love, grief, fear, and anger. After mentioning the symptoms of their diseases, and their remedies, I shall consider the morbid phenomena of joy, envy, malice, and hatred, and conclude the chapter with a few remarks upon the torpor of the passions.

Of Love

This passion, which was implanted in the human breast for the purpose of bringing the sexes together, and thereby increasing their happiness, becomes a disease only where it is disappointed in its object. The symptoms of love, when it creates disease, are, sighing, wakefulness, perpetual talking, or silence, upon the subject of the object beloved, and a predilection to solitude. Where these symptoms do not discover its existence, it may be known in a man, by blushing, and an increased frequency of pulse, when the name of the person beloved is mentioned; and in a woman, according to La Bruyere, "by her constantly looking at the man she loves when in company, or never looking at him at all." It is known further in a woman, by her retiring to decorate herself upon the appearance of the man in company whom she loves. It always renders a woman awkward, but it polishes the manners of men. The effects of unsuccessful love are dyspepsia, hysteria, hypochondriasis, fever, and madness. The last has sometimes induced suicide, while all the others have now and then ended in death.

The remedies for this disease, when accompanied with fever, or great excitement in the brain, or any other part of the system, should be,

1. Bleeding, blistering, and the other remedies for similar states of the system from other causes. It is remarkable, that persons who have been cured of the diseases from love, by these remedies, recover without feeling any affection for the persons they have loved. This was the case with one of the princes of Conde. He complained, in this state of his mind, that his physicians had drawn off all his love for his mistress by their depleting remedies.

2. Ovid advises what he calls a "binam amicam," that is, a new mistress, for unsuccessful love. I have known this remedy to succeed in several instances. The sincerity of a former attachment is often called in question, by a sudden translation of the affections to a second mistress, but without any foundation. Indeed, it proves its sincerity, for its ardour admits of no other cure.

3. The same master of the subject of love, Ovid, advises an unsuccessful lover to find out, and dwell upon all the bad qualities, and defects in person and accomplishments, of his mistress. "If she have a bad voice (says he) press her to sing; if she touch a musical instrument clumsily, beg her to expose herself by playing upon one of them."

4. The company of the person beloved should be carefully avoided. A voyage or journey should be advised in this case, for absence has been justly styled the tomb of love. The company of strangers, by checking all conversation about the person beloved, prevents the passion being cherished by it.

5. Constant employment will aid absence as a remedy for hopeless love. The more that employment interests the understanding, the more completely it will have that effect. The disease is more than half cured, when the distressed lover ceases to think of the object of his affections.

6. As hope and love are born together, so they can only die together. Uncommon pains therefore should be taken, in curing love, to extinguish every spark of hope in a lover. This advice is given with singular good sense and humanity by Dr. Gregory, in his Legacy to his Daughters, upon the subject of courtship and marriage.

7. Unsuccessful love is cured by exciting a more powerful passion in the mind. Ambition should be preferred for this purpose. Its efficacy is taken notice of by the duke of Rochefaucault. "Ambition (he says) may succeed love, but love never cures ambition."

Of Grief

Physicians, in their unsuccessful efforts to save life, are often obliged to witness this passion. It is of consequence for them, therefore, to be well acquainted with its symptoms and cure.

Its symptoms are acute and chronic. The former are, insensibility, syncope, asphyxia, and apoplexy; the latter are, fever, wakefulness, sighing, With and without tears, dyspepsia, hypochondriasis, loss of memory, gray hairs, marks of premature old age in the countenance, catalepsy, and madness. It sometimes brings on sudden death, without any signs of previous disease, either acute or chronic. Dissections of persons who have died of grief show congestion in, and inflammation of, the heart, with a rupture of its auricles and ventricles. But there are instances, in which the sympathy of the heart with the whole system is so completely dissevered by grief, that the subject of it discovers not one mark of it in his countenance or behaviour. On the contrary, he sometimes exhibits signs of unbecoming levity in his intercourse with the world. This state of mind soon passes away, and is generally followed by all the obvious and natural signs of the most poignant and durable grief.

There is another symptom of grief which is not often noticed, and that is profound sleep. I have often witnessed it even in mothers, immediately after the death of a child. Criminals, we are told by Mr. Akerman, the keeper of Newgate in London, often sleep soundly the night before their execution. The son of general Custine, slept nine hours, the night before he was led to the guillotine in Paris. These facts, and many similar ones that might be mentioned, will serve to vindicate the disciples of our Saviour from a want of sympathy with him in his suffering. They slept during his agony in the garden, because their "flesh was weak," and in consequence of "sorrow having filled their hearts."

The remedies for grief are physical, and moral. To enumerate the latter would be foreign to the design of these inquiries. They belong moreover to another profession. I shall barely glance at them, without separating them from those that are of a physical nature.

The first remedy that is indicated in recent grief is, opium. It should be given in liberal doses in its first paroxysm, and it should be repeated afterwards, in order to obviate wakefulness.

2. From the relief which the discharge of tears affords in grief, pains should be taken to procure it. The means for this purpose are, obtruding upon the mind a sorrow of a less grade than that by which it is depressed. Ancient history furnishes us with a pathetic example of the efficacy of this remedy. Psamminitus, one of the kings of Egypt, with his son, daughter and servant, were taken prisoners by Cambysis, king of Persia. Soon after his captivity, he beheld his daughter sent in the habit of a servant to draw water. This sight drew tears from his attendants, but produced no sign of distress in the king of Egypt. Immediately afterwards his son was conducted before his eyes to a

place of execution. This sight he likewise saw without an emotion of any kind. His servant next appeared before him, among a number of other captives. This sight, although accompanied with less distress than the two former, overcame him, and he suddenly burst into tears. It has been said, that "sorrows seldom come alone." The goodness of heaven is obvious in this dispensation of the evils of life; for, as sorrows generally differ in their degrees, such of them as are great, by weakening sensibility, lessen the pain from the pressure of successive lighter ones, while such as are originally light prepare the mind for the pressure of such as exceed them.

3. Should the system react, and symptoms of great excitement appear in the blood-vessels or brain, bleeding and purges should be prescribed. The latter will be rendered necessary, by the exhibition of opium.

4. The persons afflicted with grief should be carried from the room in which their relations have died, nor should they ever see their bodies afterwards. They should by no means be permitted to follow them to the grave. It would be useful to inter the body of the deceased as far as possible from the view of the person, who is the subject of grief. Graveyards in a city, and in places of public resort, are very improper, inasmuch as they either renew, and perpetuate grief, or create insensibility to death, and a criminal indifference to human dust. The patriarch Abraham understood these principles in the human heart; hence we read, when his wife died, he refused to bury her in the sepulchres of the sons of Heth, but entreated them to sell him a piece of ground, that he might "bury her out of his sight." A similar practice was adopted by the descendants of this patriarch who inhabited ancient Judea. Their grave-yards were always placed 2000 cubits from their cities. The sepulchres or vaults of the wealthy were in their gardens, which were situated in the neighbourhood of their cities. These facts will render not only more credible, but more intelligible, the account given in the New Testament of the agony of our Saviour being in a garden, near the city of Jerusalem, and his tomb, a sepulchre in which no man had laid.

The Chinese, like the Jews, inter their dead out of their cities. The Russians bury their dead after night, probably to prevent unnecessary grief,

5. As soon as the ceremonies and bustle of the funeral are over, persons afflicted with grief should be advised to receive the visits of their friends, of whom the physician should always be one. In their first visit to persons recently bereaved of their relations, they should imitate the conduct of Job's friends, who after weeping for his losses and afflictions when they beheld him afar off, the sacred historian tells us, "sat down with him upon the ground, seven days, and seven nights, and none spake a word to him, for they saw his grief was very great." Mr. Sterne has imitated, but not equalled, this delicate and affecting passage, in his history of his uncle Toby, In his first visit to his brother, after the death of his son, "he sat down (says Sterne) in an arm chair, at the head of a bed in which his brother lay, - and - said nothing."

There is science, as well as sympathy in this silence, for in this way, grief most rapidly passes from the bosom of the sufferer into that of his friend.

As soon as it is proper to begin a conversation with a person under the pressure of recent grief, such consolations should be suggested, as are offered by reason and religion. Dr. Stonehouse, the physician and friend of the pious Mr. Harvey, made it a practice to send a copy of a little work, entitled "the Mourner," written by Dr. Grovenor, to the friends of every patient he lost. It is an excellent book, and well calculated to compose the mind under this kind of affliction. A physician should listen to the history of the last stage of his patient's disease, and to the details of the appearances x>f the body after death. Much knowledge may be picked up in this way, which would otherwise perish. If any prejudice or mistake has taken place respecting his opinion of the nature of the disease of which his patient has died, or of the effects of any of his remedies, he may remove or correct them. By a visit thus paid, and employed, a physician not only wards off any complaint of his want of skill, but increases the confidence of his patients in it, and often secures their attachment to him through his subsequent life.

6. After the expiration of the weeks of mourning care should be taken never to mention the names of the deceased persons to any of their friends, nor to allude to any thing that by means of association can revive their memories. The appearance of mirth, and even cheerfulness, should be avoided. They both often give not only pain, but offence, to a mind rendered exquisitely sensible by recent grief.

Physicians are sometimes called upon to mention the deaths of relations to their patients. This should never be done at once. They should be first told that they were sick, and in great danger, and the news of their death should not be communicated until after a second or third visit.

Of Fear

There are so much danger and evil in our world, that the passion of fear was implanted in our minds for the wise and benevolent purpose of defending us from them.

The objects of fear are of two kinds,

I. Reasonable. These are, death, and surgical operations. And,

II. Unreasonable. These are, thunder, darkness, ghosts, speaking in public, sailing, riding, certain animals, particularly cats, rats, insects, and the like.

The effects of fear, when it acts suddenly upon the system, are, tremors, quick pulse and respiration, globus hystericus, a discharge of pale urine, diarrhoea, and sometimes an involuntary discharge of the faeces, aphonia, fever, convulsions, syncope, mania, epilepsy, asphyxia, death. Dr. Brambilla relates the case of a soldier, in whom fear produced not only a fever, but a mortification from a blister on the leg, which destroyed his life. Besides these general effects of fear, it acts in a peculiar manner upon the hair of the head. 1. In causing it to stand perpendicular. This has been happily described by

Virgil and Shakespeare. 2. In converting it suddenly to a gray or white colour, and 3, in causing it to come out by the roots, and to fall off the head. Of this Dr. Huch informed me he knew an instance in a gentleman who was in Lisbon, at the time of the great earthquake in 1755. .Other effects of fear have been lately noticed. The earthquake which took place on the shores of the Mississippi, in December 1811, produced silence, or great talkativeness, and moping stillness, or constant motion, in different people.

The remedies for fear are physical, rational, and moral; and here, as in the preceding chapter, I shall only hint at the moral remedies, and blend them with such as are of a rational and physical nature.

I. Of the remedies for the reasonable objects of fear.

The first object of fear under this head is death. Its remedies are,

1. Just opinions of the divine government, and of the relation we sustain to the great Author of our being. These opinions may be best formed by reading the scriptures, and such other books as derive their arguments for fortifying the mind against this fear from them, particularly the works of Dr. Sherlock and Mr. Drelincourt, both of which contain a treasure of knowledge and consolation upon this subject.

2. As much of the fear of death is produced by the dread of the pains which attend it, let us inform our patients that these pains are by no means universal, that they are less severe than the pains of many common diseases, from which there are daily recoveries, and that heaven has kindly furnished us with several remedies, which remove or mitigate them. "It is less distressing to die (says Mr. Pascall) than to think of death." This I believe is strictly true in most cases.

3. The recollection of frequent escapes from death. David met Goliah without fear, when he recollected his escapes from his conflicts with a lion and a bear. Soldiers become brave, in proportion to the number of battles they have survived.

4. The frequent meditation upon death. Dr. Horn mentions an instance of a man, who was not only cured of the fear of death by setting a portion of time every day to meditate upon it, but the subject at length became agreeable to him. In this, as well as in many other instances, painful impressions upon the mind are upon a footing with painful impressions upon the body, in being converted by repetition into such as are of a pleasurable nature.

5. Constant employment is an antidote to the fear of death; for fear, like vice, is the offspring of idleness.

6. We have an account of a method of obviating the fear of death from a public execution, in Miss Williams's history of the conduct of the marquis de Chatelet, and general Miranda, during their confinement in Paris, and at a time when they expected every day to be led to the guillotine. They read books of history and science constantly when alone, and conversed upon no other subjects when together; and although they were confined for six months in the same apartment, they never spoke to each other of their im-

pending and expected fate, by which means they lessened the fear of it. This account was confirmed to me by general Miranda, in his visit to this city a few years ago. Boys obviate fear in like manner, by silence in passing by a grave-yard, or by conversing upon subjects unconnected with death. It is not peculiar to the passion of fear to be increased by conversation. All the other passions are excited by it.

7. The fear of death is sometimes obviated by company in the last hours of life. "It is not so difficult a thing to die (said Lewis the Fourteenth, on his death bed) as I expected." Voltaire, who mentions this anecdote, endeavours to account for it, by adding, that all men die with composure or fortitude, who die in company. The courage of soldiers is derived, in a great degree, from being surrounded by persons who will bear a testimony in its favour.

8. **Music** suspends the fear of death; hence its universal use in battle. Even noise of any kind dissipates fear; hence boys obviate it not only by silence when in company, but by whistling, or hollowing when they pass by a grave - yard alone, after night.

9. **Opium** has a wonderful effect in lessening the fear of death. I have seen patients cheerful in their last moments, from the operation of this medicine upon the body and mind.

2. The fear of a surgical operation may be very much lessened by previous company, and a large dose of opium. Its pain may be mitigated by the *gradual* application of the knife, and, in tedious operations, by short intermissions in the use of it.

II. Of the unreasonable objects of fear. These are,

1. Thunder. The remedies for it are,

1. Living in a house defended by a lightning rod,

2. Sitting in the middle of a room, and remote from the doors and windows of a house, not defended by a lightning rod.

3. A citizen of Philadelphia, who was under the influence of this fear, obviated it in a degree by closing the door and windows of a room, and sitting with a lighted candle in it. By this means he avoided the sight of the lightning, and the anticipation of the noise of the thunder which usually follows it.

4. A lady of respectable character, formerly of this city, usually fainted with terror during the time of a thunder-gust, and discovered, by a livid countenance, and cold and clammy sweats, the signs of approaching death. She was apparently kept alive, by pouring into her stomach three or four wine glasses of Jamaica spirits; it was remarkable she never was intoxicated by it, and that it was disagreeable to her at all other times.

5. I crossed the Atlantic Ocean with a lady, in whom an acute head-ache was always induced by thunder. It left her as soon as the thunder ceased. Her only remedies for it were, quietness and silence. It is probable a large dose of laudanum, taken upon the appearance of a thunder-gust, would have prevented this headache, as well as obviated the terror mentioned in the two

preceding cases, more effectually than a close room artificially lighted, or a large quantity of ardent spirits.

2. The fear which is excited by darkness may easily be overcome by a proper mode of education in early life. It consists in compelling children to go to bed without a candle, or without permitting company to remain with them until they fall asleep.

3. The fear of ghosts should be prevented or subdued in early life, by teaching children the absurdity and falsehood of all the stories that are fabricated by nurses upon that subject.

4. The fear from speaking in public was always obviated by Mr. John Hunter, by taking a dose of laudanum before he met his class every day.

5. The fear from sailing, riding, and from certain animals and insects, may all be cured by resolution. It should be counteracted in early life. The existence of it always shews a defective education. Peter the Great, of Muscovy, was born with a dread of water. He cured it, by throwing himself head long into a boat when obliged to cross a river. The horror he felt in doing this often induced syncope. He finally conquered his dread of water, so as to cross seas in pursuit of the great objects which characterised his life and reign.

In cases of sudden fear from any cause, holding the breath, coughing, or hawking, often give immediate relief. They impart tone to the brain, by promoting a determination of blood to it, and thus infuse vigour into the mind.

To obviate fear from all its causes, great advantages will arise from creating counter motives in the mind. The fear of death in a battle is overcome by the powerful sense of glory, or shame. The fear of the pain of an operation, such as drawing a tooth in a child, is overcome by the expectation of receiving afterwards a piece of money, and the prospect of all the pleasures it will procure.

Great advantages may likewise be derived for the cure of fear, by a proper application of the principle of association. A horse will seldom be moved by the firing of a gun, or the beating of a drum, if he hear them for the first time while he is eating; nor will he start, or retire from a wheelbarrow, or a millstone, or any other object of that kind, after being once or twice fed upon them. The same law of association may be applied in a variety of instances to the human mind, as well to the prevention, as cure, of fear.

Of Anger

This passion was implanted in the human mind for wise and useful purposes. Its exercises, within certain limits, are admitted in the scriptures. It is only when it ascends to rage and fury, or when it is protracted into malice and revenge, that it becomes a sin and a disease.

A morbid paroxysm of anger appears in a preternatural determination of blood to the brain, a turgescence of the blood vessels of the face, a redness of the eyes, an increased secretion of saliva, which is discharged by foaming at the mouth, great volubility, or a total suppression of speech, agitations of the fists, stamping of the feet, uncommon bodily strength, convulsions, hysteria, bleeding at the nose, apoplexy, and death. Sometimes this disease appears with paleness, tremors, sickness at stomach, quick respiration, puking, syncope, and asphyxia. It is in this case generally combined with fear, and hence arises the abstraction of blood from the brain, and its determination to other parts of the body.

The remedies for anger, when it becomes a disease, divide themselves into two classes; I, such as are proper during its paroxysms; and II, such as are proper in their intervals, to prevent their recurrence.

I. To the first head belong,

1. A draught of **cold water**. This acts in two ways; 1, as a sedative; and 2, by giving time for reflection.

2. **Cold water** thrown over the whole body has in several instances cured a paroxysm of anger. It never fails to part two angry, contending dogs.

3. **Silence**. This should be observed by persons, when they are disposed to excessive anger. If this be impracticable, let the angry person repeat the Lord's prayer, or, if he be indisposed to do this, let him count twenty. The action of the organs of speech, employed in either, will serve to convey off a portion of excitement from his mind, as well as to give time for the reflux of blood from the brain.

4. The celebrated general Galvez, formerly of the Spanish army, made it a practice, when he felt himself disposed to be angry, to drink a bottle of claret. It instantly composed his mind, probably by overcoming a weak morbid action, and producing agreeable and healthy excitement in his brain. A dose of laudanum would be a better remedy for this purpose. It could not fail of being effectual in anger attended with fear, and a determination of the blood to the stomach and viscera of the thorax.

II. The means of preventing the recurrence of anger should be,

1. A milk and vegetable diet. Dr. Arbuthnot says he has seen an irascible diathesis perfectly cured by this remedy.

2. Avoiding speaking with a loud voice at all times, and especially when disposed to anger.

3. Avoiding the use of ardent and fermented liquors. They predispose to anger, even where they do not intoxicate.

4. Ballonius says, that fatigue and thirst predispose to anger. Hunger certainly has that effect. They should both therefore be carefully avoided by irascible persons.

5. Opposing to anger other passions which destroy it. Thetys, I remarked formerly, eradicated the anger of her son Achilles, by exciting in his mind the passion of love. Fear has had the same effect. The threat and the dread of a severe punishment has often prevented it in school boys and servants.

6. The cultivation of the understanding has a great influence in destroying the predisposition to anger. Science of all kinds is useful for this purpose, but the mathematics possess this property in the most eminent degree. They

produced that effect upon the temper of Sir Isaac Newton, of which the following instance is mentioned by one of his contemporaries.

Upon seeing a large collection of papers on fire that contained the calculations of many years, in consequence of his little dog jumping upon his table, and oversetting his candle upon them, he barely uttered the following words; "O! Diamond! Diamond! little dost thou know the mischief thou hast done thy master." I shall mention in another place an instance of one of his appetites being subdued in like manner, by his mind being constantly occupied by mathematical and philosophical studies. I am disposed to ascribe more to those studies than to any others, from their extending a sedative and moral influence to *all* the passions. The late Rev. Mr. Farmer, one of the ministers of the catholic church in this city, informed me, that demonstrating two or three propositions in Euclid, before he retired to his closet for the purpose of devotion, never failed to have that effect upon his mind.

7. It will be useful for persons subject to the criminal degrees of this passion, to reflect, that it is not only contrary to religion and morals, but to liberal manners. The term gentleman implies a command of this passion, above all others.

Joy

This emotion is attended sometimes with pain in the region of the heart, a change in the voice, tears, syncope, and death. Mr. Bruce mentions another symptom of excessive joy, and that is thirst, which he felt in a high degree, when he reached the long sought for head of the Nile. He gratified it, he tells us, by drinking the health of his sovereign, George the Third, and of his mistress, by a draught from the fountain of that celebrated river.

Joy is most intense, when it has been preceded by fear. The Indian Chief, Logan, has designated this form of joy in his eloquent speech, preserved by Mr. Jefferson, in his Notes upon Virginia, when he declares that "he knew not the joy of fear."

There are many instances upon record, of death being induced by a sudden paroxysm of joy. The son of the famous Leibnitz died from this cause, upon his opening an old chest, and unexpectedly finding in it a large quantity of gold. Joy, from the successful issue of political schemes or wishes, has often produced the same effect. Pope Leo the Tenth died of joy, in consequence of hearing of a great calamity that had befallen the French nation. Several persons died from the same cause, Mr. Hume tells us, upon witnessing the restoration of Charles the Second to the British throne; and it is well known the door-keeper of congress died of an apoplexy, from joy upon hearing the news of the capture of lord Cornwallis and his army, during the American revolutionary war.

During a paroxysm of joy, if it be attended with danger to life, a new emotion or passion should be excited, particularly terror, anger, fear, or grief. Perhaps the affusion of cold water might have that effect. The stimulus of artificial pain should likewise be tried. It should be of a nature calculated to produce the most prompt effects.

The morbid state of joy should be prevented, by imparting the news which we expect will create it, in a gradual manner, and with the alloy of some unpleasant circumstances.

Connected with joy, but produced by different causes, is **laughter**. It is a convulsive disease, and sometimes induces a rupture of a blood-vessel in the lungs, spleen, or brain. I have seen an instance of haemoptysis induced by it, which had a fatal issue. Two sudden deaths are upon record from it, the one of Chrysippus, an ancient Greek philosopher, the other of a pope. It was induced in the latter, while he was confined to his bed with a light indisposition, by seeing a tame monkey put on a part of his pontifical robes. Excessive laughter, when not attended with these fatal effects, is often followed with a pain in the left side, hiccup, and low spirits,

The remedies for a paroxysm of laughter should be, fear, terror, or any other counter impression. Pinching the body, or the affusion of cold water over it, is calculated to produce the same good effects. Laudanum seldom fails of relieving the pain, hiccup, and low spirits, which sometimes follow it.

Of the Morbid Effects of Envy, Malice, and Hatred

As envy is commonly the parent of malice and hatred, I shall make a few remarks upon it, and afterwards mention the combined effects of them all upon the body.

Of this vice it may be truly asserted, that it is deep seated, and always painful; hence it has been said, by an inspired writer, to resemble "rottenness in the bones;" and by Lord Bacon, "to know no holidays." It is likewise a monopolizing vice. Alexander envied his successful generals, and Garrick was hostile to all the popular players of his day. It is moreover a parricidal vice, for it not only emits its poison against its friends, but against the persons, who, by the favours it has conferred upon those who cherish it, have become in one respect the authors of their being; and, lastly, it possesses a polypus life. No kindness, gentleness, or generosity, can destroy it. On the contrary, it derives fresh strength from every act which it experienced of any of them. It likewise survives and often forgives the resentment it sometimes occasions, but without ceasing to hate the talents, virtues or personal endowments, by which it was originally excited. Nor is it satiated by the apparent extinction of them in death. This is obvious, from its so frequently opening the sanctuary of the grave, and robbing the possessors of those qualities of the slender remains it had left them of posthumous fame.

However devoid this vice and its offspring may be of remissions, they now and then appear in the form of paroxysms, which discover themselves in tremors, paleness, and a suffusion of the face with red blood. The face in this case performs the vicarious office which has lately been ascribed to the spleen. But their effects appear more frequently in slow fevers, and in a long train of nervous diseases. Persons affected with them seldom acknowledge their true cause. A single instance only of this candour is mentioned by Dr. Tissot He tells us he was once consulted by a gentleman, who told him all his complaints were brought on by his intense and habitual hatred of an enemy. Many of the chronic diseases of high life, and professional men, I have no doubt are induced by the same cause.

I once thought that medicine had not a single remedy in all its stores, that could subdue or even palliate the diseases induced by the baneful passions that have been described, and that an antidote to them was to be found only in religion; but I have since recollected one, and heard of another physical remedy, that will at least palliate them. The first is, frequent convivial society between persons who are hostile to each other. It never fails to soften resentments, and sometimes to produce reconciliation, and friendship. The reader will be surprised, when I add, that the second physical remedy was suggested to me by a madman in the Pennsylvania Hospital. In conversing with him, he produced a large collection of papers, which he said contained his Journal. "Here (said he) I write down every thing that passes in my mind, and particularly malice and revenge. In recording the latter, I feel my mind emptied of something disagreeable to it, just as a vomit empties the stomach of bile. When I look at what I have written a day or two afterwards, I feel ashamed and disgusted with it, and wish to throw it into the fire." I have no doubt of the utility of this remedy for envy, malice, and hatred, from its salutary effects in a similar case. A gentleman in this city informed me, that after writing an attack for the press upon a person who had offended him, he was so struck with its malignity, upon reading it, that he instantly destroyed it. The French nobility sometimes cover the walls and ceiling of a room in their houses with looking-glasses. The room, thus furnished, is called a Boudoir. Did ill-natured people imitate the practice of the madman and gentleman I have mentioned, by putting their envious, malicious, and revengeful thoughts upon paper, it would form a mirror, that would serve the same purpose of pointing out, and remedying, the evil dispositions of the mind, that the boudoirs in France serves, in discovering and remedying the detects in the attitudes and dress of the body.

To persons who are not ashamed, nor disgusted, with the first sight of their malevolent effusions upon paper, the same advice may be given, that Dr. Franklin gave to a gentleman, who read part of a humorous satire which he had written upon the person and character of a respectable citizen of Philadelphia. After he had finished reading it, he asked the Doctor what he thought of his publishing it? "Keep it by you, said the Doctor, for one year, and then ask me that question." The gentleman felt the force of this answer, and went immediately to the printer, who had composed the first page of it, took it from him, and consigned the whole manuscript to oblivion.

I shall conclude the history of the passions, by remarking, that their symptoms, and force, are varied by a difference in predisposition, age, rank in society, profession, moral and religious habits, duration, and by their acting singly, or in combination with each other.

There is now and then a **torpor of the passions,** the reverse of the diseases in them which have been described. Instead of being unduly excited, they are devoid of all sensibility and irritability. Persons who are thus affected love and fear nothing. They are strangers to grief and anger; they envy and hate nobody; and they are alike insensible to mental pleasure and pain. I was once consulted by a citizen of Philadelphia, who was remarkable for his strong affection for his wife and children when his mind was in a sound state, who was occasionally afflicted with this apathy, and when under its influence lost his affection for them all, so entirely, that he said he could see them butchered before his eyes without feeling any distress, or even an inclination to rise from his chair to protect them.

This paralytic state of all the passions continues during life in some people: a physician of great eminence, who died some years ago in England, declared, upon his death bed, that he had never known what it was to love man, woman, or child. But we sometimes meet with this *disorder* in a partial state. Thus are there men who have never loved, others who have never feared, others who have never shed a tear, and others in whom no injuries have ever excited an emotion of anger. In such persons, the mind is in a mutilated state; for man, without all his passions, is an imperfect being, both as to his duties and happiness.

The remedies for this torpid state of the passions, whether general or partial, should be suited to the state of the system. Depletion will be proper, if the blood-vessels are oppressed. In a contrary state of the system, powerful stimulants, particularly pain, labour, the cold bath, and a salivation are indicated. I mentioned formerly an instance in which mercury restored the affection of a mother for her child in a day or two after it affected her mouth.

Chapter Eighteen - Of the Morbid state of the Sexual Appetite

His appetite, which was implanted in our natures for the purpose of propagating our species, when excessive, becomes a disease both of the body and mind. When restrained, it produces tremors, a flushing of the face, sighing, nocturnal pollutions, hysteria, hypochondriasis, and in women the furor uterinus. When indulged in an undue or a promiscuous intercourse with the female sex, or in onanism, it produces seminal weakness, impotence, dysury, tabes dorsalis, pulmonary consumption, dyspepsia, dimness of sight, vertigo, epilepsy, hypochondriasis, loss of memory, manalgia, fatuity, and death. From a number of letters addressed to me, for advice, I shall select but three, in which many of those symptoms are mentioned, and deplored in the most pathetic terms. The first is from a physician in Massachusetts, dated September 4th, 1793.

"The gentleman whose case is now submitted to you is about twenty-five years of age, meagre, gloomy, and restless, has a bad countenance, and a lax state of bowels. He imputes his indisposition to his excessive devotedness to Venus, which he thinks has been induced by a morbid state of his body. He has been married three years, had no connection with the sex before he married, and, although he feels disgusted with his strong venereal propensities, he cannot resist them. I advised him to separate himself from his wife by travelling, which he did, but without experiencing any relief from his disease. He has earnestly requested me to render him impotent, if I could not give him the command of himself in any other way. I have tried several remedies in his case; nothing has done him any good except the sugar of lead, which I was soon obliged to lay aside, from its producing a severe nervous cholic. Wishing to know whether his disease was not seated in his imagination only, I asked whether the gratification of his appetite was equal to his desires. Dixit, per annos tres, quinque vices se coitum fecisse in horis viginti quatuor, et semper semine ejecto."

The second letter, to which I have alluded, is from the miserable subject of the disease that is described in it. After acknowledging its cause to be from onanism, he adds, "I rest badly at nights, and am much troubled with dreams. I have frequent nocturnal erections, accompanied with a sensation of uneasiness, instead of desire or pleasure; and from dreams, frequent emissions take place, which are much more fluid than natural. The external organs of generation have a numb, or dead, feeling. The lower part of my back is weak; my eyes are often painful and my eye-lids swelled and red. I have an almost constant cold, and oppression at my stomach. In short, I had rather be laid in the silent tomb, and encounter that dreadful uncertainty, *hereafter,* than remain in my present unhappy and degraded situation. These are humiliating concessions, and it is extremely painful for me to make them; but let my melancholy situation be my apology for them."

The third and last letter upon this subject is from a physician in Virginia, in which he describes the disease of a patient then under his care, in the following words. "A. B. aged seventeen, of a cold phlegmatic temperament of body, of a sedentary life, and studious habits, in consequence of indulging in the solitary vice of onanism, has lately become very much diseased. His vision is indistinct, and his memory much impaired, and he now labours under much muscular relaxation, prostration of strength, atrophy, and depression of spirits. His system is so very irritable, that the least agitation of mind, or riding on horseback, or gently rubbing his breast, or even combing his hair, seminis emissionem inducunt. Any plan you may suggest for the relief of this truly wretched being will be gratefully received."

But these are not all the melancholy and disgusting effects of excess in the indulgence of the sexual appetite. They sometimes discover themselves in the imagination and senses, in a fondness for obscene conversation and books, and in a wanton dalliance with women, long after the ability to gratify the appetite has perished from disease, or age.

The remote and exciting causes of this disease in the sexual appetite are,

1. Excessive eating, more especially of high seasoned animal food. The vices of the cities of the plain were denied in part from their "fulness of bread;" by which is meant an excess of nourishing aliment.

2. Intemperance in drinking. Hence the frequent transition from the bottle to the brothel! It is because it is so common and natural, that the former is generally mentioned as an apology for the disease contracted in the latter, by young men, in their application to physicians for remedies for it. The incestuous gratification of the sexual appetite, which was the first sin that revived in the world after the flood, was the effect we are told of the intemperate use of wine.

3. Idleness. This was another of the causes mentioned in the Old Testament of the vices of the cities of the plain. It is from the effects of indolence and sedentary habits that the venereal appetite prevails with so much force, and with such odious consequences, within the walls of those seminaries of learning, in which a number of young men are herded together, and lodge in the same rooms, or in the same beds.

The remedies for this appetite, when inordinate, are natural, physical and mental. They are,

1. Matrimony; but where this is not practicable, the society of chaste and modest women. While men live by themselves (says La Bruere) they do not view washerwomen or oyster-wenches as washerwomen or oyster wenches, but simply as women. But by mixing with the sex, they lose the habit of associating the idea of the sex of the women with a cap or a petticoat. I have known few young men of loose morals, who have attached themselves to the society of the ladies. They not only polish their manners, but purify their imaginations.

2. A diet, consisting simply of vegetables, and prepared without any of the usual condiments that are taken with them. Dr. Stark found his venereal desires nearly extinguished by living upon bread and water. They revived upon a diet of bread and milk, and became more active by eating six or eight ounces of roasted goose every day, with a proportionable quantity of bread. Persons afflicted with this disease should use but little salt in their aliment. Plutarch tells us, it was avoided by the priests in his day, from its disposing to venery. The birth of Venus from the sea was probably intended to signify the connection between the use of salt and the venereal appetite. In recommending a vegetable diet for the cure of this disease, I would remark, that it is effectual only when it *succeeds* a full animal diet; for we read not only of individuals, but of whole nations, that live upon vegetables and other simple food, in whom the sexual appetite exists in its usual and natural force. In such persons the appetite should be weakened, by reducing the *quantity* of their aliment.

3. Temperance in drinking, or rather the total abstinence from all fermented and distilled liquors.

4. Constant employment in bodily labour or exercise. They both lessen venereal excitability and promote healthy excitement. Hippocrates tells us the Sythians, who nearly lived upon horseback, were free from venereal desires. Long journeys on horseback should therefore be recommended for the morbid degrees of this appetite. The chase would probably serve the same purpose. The connection between this exercise and chastity is happily illustrated by the poets in the character of Diana, who lived by hunting. The Indians owe the weakness of their venereal desires to this, among other invigorating employments.

5. The cold bath. There is a debility of body which is connected with venereal excitability, and which the cold bath is calculated to remove. This excitability is most apt to occur during the convalescence, or soon after the recovery from malignant or chronic fevers. Twelve marriages took place of the patients who recovered from the yellow fever at Bush-Hill, in the neighbourhood of this city, in the year 1793; and a greater number were detected in a criminal intercourse with each other, in the private apartments and tents belonging to the hospital. I have known two instances of young clergymen, who married the women who nursed them in chronic fevers, both of whom were in very humble life. The celebrated Mr. Howard did the same thing. These unequal matches appear to have been the effects of a morbid sexual appetite, that suddenly succeeded their fevers, and which they did not dare to gratify but in a lawful way.

6. A salivation, by diverting morbid excitability from the genitals to the mouth and throat, would probably be useful in this disease.

7. Avoiding all dalliance with the female sex. I knew a gentleman in this city, who assured me he had gained a complete victory over his venereal desires by a strict regard to this direction; and I have heard of a clergyman, who overcame this appetite by never looking directly in the face of a woman.

3. Avoiding the sight of obscene pictures, the reading obscene books, and listening to obscene conversation, all of which administer fuel to the sexual appetite.

9. Certain tones of music have sometimes suddenly relieved a paroxysm of venereal desires.

10. Dr. Boerhaave says a sudden fit of laughter has sometimes had the same effect.

11. Close application of the mind to business, or study of any kind, more especially to the mathematics. Sir Isaac Newton conquered this appetite by means of the latter study, and the late Dr. Fothergill by constant application to business. Both these great and good men lived and died bachelors, and both declared, upon their death beds, that they never had known, in a single instance, a criminal connection with the female sex.

12. The influence of an active passion, that shall predominate over the sexual appetite. The love of military glory, so common among the American Indians, by combining with the hardships of a savage life, contributes very much to weaken their venereal desires.

13. Several medicines have been recommended, to subdue the excess of the sexual appetite; among these, the castor oil nut, and camphor, have been most commended. The former acts only by opening the bowels, and thereby taking off the tension of the contiguous genital organs. Any other lenient purge would probably have the same effect. If camphor have any virtues, in this disease, it must be by its stimulating powers removing that nervous debility, upon which venereal excitability depends. Any other stimulating medicine, given in a similar state of the system, would probably have the same, or a greater, effect.

I have thus mentioned all the remedies for derangement in the passions and sexual appetite. While I admit the necessity of their being aided by religious influence, in order to render them successful, I maintain that religious influence is seldom effectual for that purpose, unless it be combined with those physical remedies. This opinion is amply supported by numerous precepts in the Old and New Testaments, and it is only by inculcating those physical precepts, with such as are of a religious and moral nature, that the latter can produce their full effects upon the body and mind.

Chapter Nineteen - Of Derangement in the Moral Faculties

I took notice formerly of moral derangement in the will, and mentioned its symptoms, as they appeared in several specific vices. This disease discovers itself only in the moral faculty, and exists with a sound state of the conscience and sense of deity. Under the present head, I shall make a few remarks upon moral derangement, as it appears in all those moral faculties of the mind.

For an account of the nature and offices of the moral faculty and conscience, and of the difference between them, the reader is referred to an oration delivered by the author before the American Philosophical Society, in the year 1786, and published in the first volume of his Medical Inquiries and Observations. For proofs of the existence of an innate sense of deity in the human mind, the reader is referred to lord Kaims' Sketches of the History of Man. All these faculties are liable to derangement, partially and universally.

I. *Partial* derangement in them is sometimes Induced,

1. By ardent spirits.

2. By famine, the effects of which in annihilating the obligations, not only of morality, but of consanguinity, and inducing the grossest acts of cruelty are recorded in the 56th and 57th verses of the 28th chapter of Deuteronomy.

The consonance of the prediction contained in those verses with the state of the human mind, in similar circumstances of distress from hunger, has been established in many instances, in the histories of crews who have sought relief from shipwreck in a boat, or on a desolate shore.

II. The moral faculty, conscience, and the sense of deity, are sometimes *totally* deranged. The duke of Sully has given us a striking instance of this universal moral derangement, in the character of a young man who belonged to his suit, of the name of Servin, who, after a life uncommonly distinguished by every possible vice, died, cursing and denying his God. Mr. Halsam has described two cases of it in the Bethlehem Hospital, one of whom, a boy of thirteen years of age, was perfectly sensible of his depravity, and often asked, "why God had not made him like other men." He was, as might be expected, completely miserable, and often expressed a wish for death. An epitome of all that has been recorded, or perhaps seen, of this derangement in the moral faculties has been given by Edgar of himself, in the tragedy of King Lear, in the following lines.

> "I was a serving man, proud in heart and mind,
> That served the lust of my mistress' heart,
> And did the act of darkness with her;
> Swore as many oaths as I spake words;
> Wine I lov'd deeply, dice dearly:
> I was false of heart, light of ear, and bloody of hand;
> Hog in filth, fox in stealth, wolf in greediness,
> Dog in madness, and lion in prey."

In the course of my life, I have been consulted in three cases of the total perversion of the moral faculties. One of them was in a young man, the second in a young woman, both of Virginia, and the third was in the daughter of a citizen of Philadelphia. The last was addicted to every kind of mischief. Her wickedness had no intervals while she was awake, except when she was kept busy in some steady and difficult employment. In all these cases of innate, preternatural moral depravity, there is probably an original defective organization in those parts of the body, which are occupied by the moral faculties of the mind.

How far the persons whose diseases have been mentioned, should be considered as responsible to human or divine laws for their actions, and where the line should be drawn that divides free agency from necessity, and vice from disease, I am unable to determine. In whatever manner this question may be settled, it will readily be admitted that such persons are, in a pre-eminent degree, objects of compassion, and that it is the business of medicine to aid both religion and law, in preventing and curing their moral alienation of mind. We are encouraged to undertake this enterprise of humanity, by the sameness of the laws which govern the body and the moral faculties of man. I shall venture to point out the sameness of those laws in a few instances, by mentioning the predisposition and proximate causes, the symptoms, and the remedies of corporeal and moral diseases.

1. Is debility the predisposing cause of disease in the body? so it is of vice in the mind. This debility in the mind consists in indolence, or a want of occupation. Bunyan has justly said, in support of this remark, that "an idle man's brain is the devil's work shop." The young woman, whose moral derangement I mentioned a little while ago, was always inoffensive when she was busy. The employment contrived for her by her parents was, to mix two or three papers of pins of different sizes together, and afterwards, to oblige her to separate, and sort them. The near relation of debility and vice has been expressed by the schoolmen in the following words "non posse, est *malum* posse." To do nothing, is generally to do evil.

2. Do we prevent disease, by removing the body out of the way of its exciting causes acting upon debility? In like manner, we prevent vice, by removing the mind, in its debilitated state, out of the way of bad company, and thus abstract it from the stimulus of vicious motives upon the will.

3. Does bodily disease consist in morbid excitement, or irregular action? Vice consists in like manner in undue excitement of the passions and will, and in their irregular, or, to use a scriptural epithet, in their "crooked" actions.

4. Is bodily disease a unit? So is vice. All its innumerable forms are derived simply from inordinate self-love.

5. Do high degrees of morbid bodily excitement require depleting remedies? High degrees of vice require remedies of a similar nature, such as the abstraction of company, and the excessive or criminal gratification of the passions and senses.

6. Do we overcome morbid action in a bodily disease in a highly vital part, by exciting it in a part less essential to life? In like manner we cure the odious vice of avarice, and a debasing love of pleasure, by the less odious and debasing vice of ambition.

7. Is it impossible to produce two sensations of unequal force, at the same time, in the body? It is equally impossible for the mind to act under the impression of two motives at the same time. Hence the truth of that declaration of our Saviour, "that no man can serve two masters, that is, God and Mammon." The predominance of the motive excited by one of them, will always destroy the others.

8. Do we accommodate stimuli to the state of excitability in diseases of the body? The same thing is done in all the successful applications of moral stimuli, or motives, to the will. Our Saviour hints at this accommodation of moral remedies to the peculiar state of the mind, when he alludes to the practice of not putting new wine, full of an active fermenting principle, into old bottles, which in ancient Judea, were made of leather, and of course, became weak from age.

9. Is the excessive morbid excitement of a disease worn down by labour? Excessive vicious excitement is reduced in like manner by the same means, and, in addition to it, by solitude, shame, and certain restraints or pains inflicted upon the body, of a nature calculated to act indirectly upon the mind. I acknowledge the first impressions of confinement and bodily pain generally produce a vicious fretfulness, and sometimes impious expressions and immoral conduct; but these effects of those moral remedies are generally very transient. When continued long enough, they never fail of producing a change in the moral temper of the mind. A remarkable instance of the truth of this remark occurred some years ago in the jail of Philadelphia. A notorious offender amused himself, for some time after his confinement, by drawing pictures, and writing verses of a ludicrous nature, upon the walls of his solitary cell. At the end of several weeks he became silent and pensive, and at the same time the following passage of scripture, written by him, was discovered upon one of the walls of his cell. "Come unto me, all ye who labour and are heavy laden, and I will give you rest."

10. Are bodily sensibility and irritability weakened, or destroyed, by the protracted application of morbid stimuli to sensible and irritable parts? The same thing takes place from the long application of vicious impressions to the moral faculties of the mind. They become, in such cases, to use the words of one of the apostles, "dead," and "seared with a red hot iron." A disease resembling a palsy affects them all.

I might go on further, and mention, more particularly, the analogy between bodily and moral diseases, and the propriety of adapting specific remedies to specific vices; but enough I hope has been said to show the truth and importance of the subject, and the practicability of the undertaking, by persons whose professional studies and employment are more nearly related to it than the author's. However useful the rational and physical remedies that have been mentioned may be to prevent or cure vice, they never can perform that work completely, without the aid of that supernatural and mysterious remedy which it hath pleased God to unite with them in his moral government of his creatures, and that is, the **forgiveness** of it. In vain have legislators substituted the exterminating axe and halter, and the influence of ignominious or painful corporeal punishments, for this divine mode of curing moral evil. The danger and mortality of the venereal disease were encreased, in former times, by the contempt, neglect, and corporeal chastisement, to which persons affected with it were exposed. Since the pain and shame of the disease have been considered as its ample punishments, and the subjects of it restored to public favour, the disease has every where declined, and is now rarely attended with danger, or the loss of life. The abolition of the punishment of death, and of cropping, branding, and public whipping, and substituting for them, confinement, labour, simple diet, cleanliness, and affectionate treatment, as means of reformation and forgiveness, have produced similar moral effects in the jail of Philadelphia. If this original and humane institution, in which science and relish have blended their resources together, has not been attended with uniform success, it must be ascribed wholly to the imperfect manner with which the principles that suggested it have been carried into effect. They have been rendered abortive, chiefly, by the criminals sleeping in the same room, and by the facility and frequency with which pardons are obtained for them. The former prevents the resuscitation of conscience, and all moral and religious reflection. The latter is opposed to the great axioms upon which the penal law of Pennsylvania is founded; that "punishments should be certain, but not severe, and that a pardoning power should not be lodged in any department of a government."

May this Christian system of criminal jurisprudence spread, without any of its imperfections, throughout the world! and may the rulers of nations learn from it, that the reformation of criminals, as well as the prevention of crimes, should be the objects of all punishments, and that the latter can be effected much better by living than by dead examples!

Here the reader and the author must take leave of each other. Before I retire from his sight, I shall only add, if I have not advanced, agreeably to my wishes, the interests of medicine by this work, I hope my labours in the cause of humanity will not be alike unsuccessful; and that the sufferings of our fellow creatures, from the causes that have been mentioned, may find sympathy in the bosoms, and relief from the kindness, of every person who shall think it worth while to read this history of them.

www.ingramcontent.com/pod-product-compliance
Lightning Source LLC
Chambersburg PA
CBHW022113280326
41933CB00007B/374